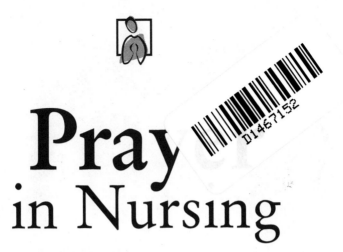

Prayer
in Nursing

The Spirituality of
Compassionate Caregiving

Prayer
in Nursing

The Spirituality of
Compassionate Caregiving

Mary Elizabeth O'Brien, SFCC
PHD, MTS, RN, FAAN

The Catholic University of America
School of Nursing

JONES AND BARTLETT PUBLISHERS
Sudbury, Massachusetts
BOSTON   TORONTO   LONDON   SINGAPORE

World Headquarters
Jones and Bartlett Publishers
40 Tall Pine Drive
Sudbury, MA 01776
978-443-5000
info@jbpub.com
www.jbpub.com

Jones and Bartlett Publishers Canada
2406 Nikanna Road
Mississauga, ON L5C 2W6
CANADA

Jones and Bartlett Publishers International
Barb House, Barb Mews
London W6 7PA
UK

Library of Congress Cataloging-in-Publication Data not available at time of printing.

ISBN: 0-7637-2239-1

Acquisitions Editor: Penny M. Glynn
Production Manager: Amy Rose
Associate Production Editor: Tara McCormick
Editorial Assistant: Karen Zuck
Production Assistant: Karen C. Ferreira
Senior Marketing Manager: Alisha Weisman
Marketing Associate: Joy Stark-Vancs
Manufacturing and Inventory Coordinator: Amy Bacus
Cover Design: Kristin E. Ohlin
Composition: Chiron, Inc.
Printing and Binding: Malloy, Inc.
Cover Printing: Malloy, Inc.

Printed in the United States of America
06 05 04 03 02   10 9 8 7 6 5 4 3 2 1

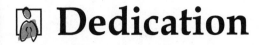 # Dedication

For all nurses who strive through prayer to practice the art and science of compassionate caregiving.

Also by Mary Elizabeth O'Brien:

Spirituality in Nursing: Standing on Holy Ground, Second Edition

Publishing in 2003:

Parish Nursing

Contents

Introduction

On a number of occasions, both colleagues and students have asked if I knew of a book of prayers, or a book about prayer, for nurses. My answer, in terms of contemporary publications, was negative. Several times an inquirer's response has been, "Why don't you write one?" The problem is that I do not feel I really know how to pray; or, at best, I am a rank amateur at the effort. And yet, I love and value prayer deeply; in fact, I have come to learn that I can't function without it. So, after a significant amount of *prayer*, I decided that I would attempt to explore the meaning of prayer for nurses. The following pages reflect the results of my study and, most importantly, my prayer.

I need to begin by noting that just as nursing is a practice-discipline, prayer is a practice-activity. You can only learn so much about it from this book, or from any other book for that matter; the real learning about prayer comes in the doing. The great thing about prayer, however, is that while you are practicing, you are also positively influencing your spiritual well-being. Does it always feel that way? Perhaps not, especially in the beginning, but that is the beautiful and mysterious thing about prayer. It's something we do, but the grace to pray is a unique gift of God. It may take a while to get the wrappings off our present, which can be frustrating. But once we begin to glimpse the treasure inside, the beauty of God's love and closeness in our lives, we know, truly, that we have found a proverbial "pearl of great price."

What should a book *of prayers* and *about prayer* for nurses contain? First, it is important to look at our spiritual heritage, the history of prayer in nursing, as well as to explore the importance of prayer for the contemporary caregiver, all of which are covered in the first chapter. Another goal of the introductory chapter is to identify and describe the charism of nursing—prayerful devotion to caring for the sick. In Chapter 2, prayer is related to the nurse's vocation, envisioned as a "holy" calling, and the present-day relevance of the Nightingale Pledge is explored through the process of spiritual retrieval. Chapter 3 examines how a nurse may discern God's will through prayerful listening to the Holy Spirit, supported by reading the Holy Scripture. In Chapter 4, I focus on caring nurse-patient relationships, relating these relationships to the nurse's prayer covenant with God. Chapter 5 examines the topic of compassion as related to a nurse's prayer life. The aim of Chapter 6 is to investigate the role of emotions in relation to prayer, especially in times of dryness or other forms of suffering. Chapter 7 explores the connection between prayer and a healing ministry, employing as an historical prefigure the nurse healer Veronica, who legend teaches wiped the face of Jesus on his journey to the Calvary; also included in Chapter 7 is a meditative "Way of the Cross" for nurses. Chapter 8 concludes the discussion of prayer in nursing by examining mental prayer in a variety of forms, including meditation, centering prayer, and contemplation. This chapter also identifies a number of spiritual writers whose works may help to support and facilitate a nurse's developing prayer life. In this concluding chapter, the topic of contemplative nursing is discussed; a serious prayer life is presented as possible and necessary for contemporary nurses seeking to practice compassion in the carrying out of their therapeutic activities. To provide some prayerful thoughts that may be helpful for nurses to consider either as individuals or in groups, each chapter begins with a nursing meditation and ends with a nurse's prayer, both of which are related to the theme of that chapter.

Acknowledgements

I wish to express my prayerful gratitude to colleagues and friends who critiqued early drafts of the present work. Faye G. Abdellah, EdD, ScD, FAAN, carefully and caringly evaluated the work for its relevance to the spiritual needs of practicing nurses; Elizabeth McFarlane, DNSc, FAAN, painstakingly reviewed the manuscript in light of her personal spirituality of nursing; Joseph J. Scott, CSP, was unfailingly available to listen, to guide, and to provide a gentle "cheering squad" when needed; and nurse practitioners Bonnie B. Benetato, FNP; Cynthia M. Cordova, MSN; and Cynthia Grandjean, CANP, provided responses to the prayers and meditations included in the text. I am also deeply appreciative of the work of Penny Glynn, RN, PhD; Karen Zuck; Karen Ferreira; Joy Stark-Vancs; and Amy Rose of Jones and Bartlett Publishers for enthusiastically and caringly shepherding the manuscript to publication.

Ultimately, my greatest gratitude is to God, the source of my strength and the center of my life. To the Father who guides my steps with His Word, to the Divine Son whose love nourishes my soul, and to the Holy Spirit who inspires and mentors my thoughts, I give loving and reverent thanks.

1 ⬛ Prayer in Nursing: Reclaiming Our Spiritual Heritage

"Pray without ceasing."
1 Thessalonians 5: 17

COMPASSIONATE CAREGIVING: THE PRACTICE OF PRAYER IN NURSING

Sitting humbly amidst His followers, on a Galilean hillside,
He taught of compassionate caregiving;
The Carpenter of Nazareth, the Lamb of God, the
Savior of the world,
who promised:
"Whatever you do for my least ones,
you do for me!"

His lesson is so simple;
His message so caring:
give some food to those who are hungry;
give a drink to someone who's thirsty;
welcome strangers;
dress people who need clothes;
visit your brothers and sisters who can't
get out;
and
take care of the sick.

"I've not had as much time as I'd like to pray lately, Dear God,"
a geriatric nurse whispers, as she tenderly lifts a spoonful
of soup to the lips of a frail elder.

"Dear Lord, if only I could fit more scripture reading into my
life," an ICU nurse prays, as he solicitously places some ice
chips on the parched tongue of a newly extubated patient.

1

*"I'd love to spend more hours in church with You, Dear Lord," an ER nurse
implores, as she compassionately helps a homeless stranger onto a waiting
gurney.*

*"Dear Lord, even when I pray I sometimes feel far away from You,"
    a recovery room nurse admits, as he caringly piles warm
    blankets on a shivering post-op patient.*

*"I want to visit with You much more in prayer, Dear Lord," a home
    care nurse muses, as she lovingly comforts a disabled patient
    in his loneliness.*

*"Dear God, I wish I knew how to pray better," a hospital staff
    nurse longs, as he gently wraps a blood-pressure cuff around
    the trembling arm of a new admission.*

*The Lord replies to His nurses: "I treasure your desire for
    intimacy with me;
                it must always be so,
                    but
                remember also
                    that*

*I am the hungry elder to whom you tenderly feed a cup of soup;
I am the thirsty ICU patient whose parched tongue you
    solicitously moisten;
I am the homeless stranger you compassionately welcome to your
    ER;
I am the shivering post-op patient you caringly clothe;
I am the homebound person you lovingly visit;
        and,
It is my trembling arm round which you gently wrap your blood-
        pressure cuff.*

*It is I, dear nurse, for whom you care, and in that caring,
    your nursing is blessed with the gift of My Presence.
            In that caring,
        your nursing becomes your prayer;
                and
            I accept it with joy."*

THE HOMELESS PATIENT: A PARABLE OF NURSING COMPASSION

It was Saturday night at the city hospital where I supervised, and the emergency room was hopping. I'd never personally worked the ER, but after a plaintive call for help from the charge nurse, I decided to grab my pager and enter the fray – at least until a more competent nursing temp could be found to assist the staff.

Arriving at the admissions desk, I asked the harried unit clerk what I could do to help. "Well," she said, "there's this homeless man in room 3. I mean, I guess he's homeless; he certainly looks it. You know, ragged clothes, long hair and beard, kind of like a sixties hippie. I didn't really get much out of him. But," she added, "somebody definitely beat him up. The police found him falling down in the street and brought him in. Maybe you could check him out and," she concluded raising a skeptical eyebrow, "find out if he really belongs here!"

As I drew back the curtain in room 3, I saw that the clerk had accurately described our latest admission. He was stretched out on a gurney dressed in worn sandals, faded jeans, and a threadbare sweatshirt; his hands were tucked, monklike, into the front pocket of his pullover. His hair was held in place by a frayed bandanna wrapped around his forehead and tied in the back.

The patient opened his eyes and smiled weakly as I approached the bed. I tried a barrage of questions: "Sir, could you tell me your name? Do you know where you are? Can you remember what happened to you?" He simply nodded serenely and said: "They beat me; they didn't know what they were doing." "Are you in pain?" I asked anxiously. "I'm thirsty," he replied. I brought him a large glass of juice, which he eagerly gulped through the straw I held for him. He kept his hands hidden; "probably doesn't want me to see the needle tracks that would identify him as an addict," I guessed.

His vital signs were stable, and his color improved markedly after downing both a second and third large glass of juice. He sat up slowly and said: "I think I can leave now; I'm feeling better. I'm just so very tired." "I wish I could let you sleep here," I responded sadly, "but we're really busy." I hastily added, "I'm sure the shelter down the street will put you up for the night." "I understand," he replied, kindly.

I put my arm around his shoulders and carefully helped him off the gurney. As he stood up, he gazed at me with the most piercing and the most tender look I have ever seen, and said, "I'll always remember how you cared for me." As he spoke the words, he removed his hands from the

sweatshirt and gently grasped my own between them. That's when I saw
his scars; not the needle marks I had almost expected but the nail holes, I
had almost missed. My Lord and my God!

As both the meditation on compassionate caregiving and the
parable of nursing compassion illustrate, the ordinary, everyday tasks
of nursing may take on a dimension of prayer for the caregiver; this is
the blessing of the nurse's calling. There are times, however, when in the
course of our nursing activities, we are called upon to enter into a place of
more conscious prayer; these occasions also constitute a blessing for the
nurse. I remember one such occurrence vividly:

"Will you say a prayer for Beth?" the mother of a 16-year-old lymphoma patient begged, her eyes pleading for a remission or, at least, for a
respite from the vicious side effects of the chemotherapy. "Of course, I'll
pray with you," I responded, admittedly with more bravado in my voice
than in my heart. It was not, surely, that I did not want to pray for this
desperately ill teen, whom I had come to both admire and love during
her many hospitalizations. Beth was gentle and kind, and unfailingly
courageous, despite her suffering; she was also dying, and it was breaking the hearts of those of us who cared for her. My reticence about the
request to pray dealt only with my personal shyness in the arena of verbal
prayer. I believe that I, as all nurses, desire to have practice skills well
honed to meet the needs of patients and families. But, of course, there is
no nursing exam we can sit for, no credentialing we can seek, which will
certify us in the art and practice of prayer.

So, as on a number of occasions past, I silently sought the guidance
of the Lord, who alone truly knows our needs and understands our
hearts. I prayed for the gift of prayer in that moment, that the words I
might speak would be His words and not mine, and that the thoughts I
might express would come from His tender care and not my own. I asked
to be an instrument, to be used, as the great St. Teresa of Avila taught, that
I might touch with His compassion the immense fragility of this precious
young spirit.

In a small but powerful book on prayer, Benedictine Mary Clare
Vincent observed "a life without prayer doesn't work."[1] I would add that
nursing without prayer doesn't work. For contemporary nurses, prayer
is, I believe, more necessary to support their caring for the sick than in any
preceding era. Complex moral and ethical issues, related both directly
and tangentially to our practice, abound in the current world of health
care. Therapeutic procedures involving a variety of extraordinary
measures to prolong human life (some of which are admittedly positive)

become more sophisticated each year; and medical research on such frightening issues as cloning of human beings hovers on the fringe of acceptable medical discourse in certain quarters.

If, in fact, we subscribe to the spiritual vision of our profession's founder, how can we not believe in the importance and value of prayer for a nurse? For it was Florence Nightingale who reminded us, in the late nineteenth century, that "God's precious gift of life is often placed literally in [the nurse's] hands."[2] What a sacred commission Nightingale issued to her followers — to hold in our hands "God's precious gift of life." How can we be faithful to such a blessed ministry without the grace of prayer? And yet, in this era of health care reform, of managed care and restructured nursing roles, what does prayer mean for the contemporary nurse? How can time for prayer be found in a caregiving system in which all activities must be cost effective, as mandated by the institutions in which we carry out our nursing activities? The purpose of this book is to address these and related questions and concerns for present day nurses; the ultimate goal is to explore the practice of prayerful, compassionate caregiving in the world of twenty-first-century nursing.

RECLAIMING OUR SPIRITUAL HERITAGE: A HISTORY OF PRAYER IN NURSING

From its inception, nursing the sick has been considered a vocation or calling; in the early days, especially, nursing was viewed as a ministry of God and of His Church and was guided and strengthened by the prayer of the caregiver. Our nursing forebears, on whose strong shoulders we contemporary nurses stand, understood this calling; they responded by including prayer as a central and critical component of their nursing ministries. In the book *Spirituality in Nursing: Standing on Holy Ground*, I devoted an entire chapter to the spiritual history of nursing. Tales of nursing prefigures from the early deacons and deaconesses of the first century, through the medieval monastics such as Hildegard of Bingen and St. Francis of Assisi, up to members of the post-reformation religious orders, are replete with anecdotes indicating the prayerfulness with which nursing ministries were undertaken.[3] For these men and women, committed to a religious vocation of caring for the sick, God's call, heard in prayer, not only was the incentive for undertaking the ministry but also was the very fiber from which a daily tapestry of nursing activities was woven.

Despite the fairly comprehensive body of writing on the spiritual history of nursing, I did not have any clear direction as to how to specifically explore the topic of prayer in nursing from a historical perspective. After praying to the Holy Spirit for guidance, I decided that I would camp out for a time in a wonderfully prayerful place in our Catholic University nursing library, the Mary Walsh Room. The Mary Walsh Room is a cozy, graciously appointed space hidden away in a back corner of the library; its floor-to-ceiling bookshelves are crammed from end to end with a magnificent collection of books documenting the history of professional nursing. The collection also contains bound volumes of early periodicals such as *The American Journal of Nursing, The Trained Nurse and Hospital Review, The Public Health Nurse,* and *The Catholic Nurse.*

I spent a significant portion of one summer ensconced in a comfy chair in the Mary Walsh Room perusing books and periodicals in search of references to prayer in the history of our profession. I delighted in numerous "finds," documenting the importance and centrality of prayer in the personal and professional lives of our early nurses; and I discovered, joyfully, that prayer has been extensively practiced and deeply valued by nurses since the era of our founder, Florence Nightingale. The fruits of my research are interwoven throughout discussions of prayer in the present and following chapters.

As early as the mid-nineteenth century, Florence Nightingale's life and writings modeled a variety of prayers. In a letter to her Aunt Hannah, written in 1846, Florence described her prayer of petition: "I never pray for anything temporal . . . but when each morning comes, I kneel down before the Rising Sun and only say: 'Behold the handmaid of the Lord, give me this day my work to do, no, not my work, but Thine.'"[4] A Nightingale diary entry acknowledges the author's listening to the Lord in prayer: "God called me in the morning and asked me: 'Would I do good for Him, for Him alone without reputation [self-interest].'"[5] Florence's mystical bent and her gift for contemplation are reflected in a famous quote from *Notes for Devotional Authors*: "Where shall I find God? In myself. That is the true mystical doctrine. But then I myself must be in a state for Him to come and dwell in me."[6]

In a letter to a cherished mentor and friend, Dr. Benjamin Jowett, Florence articulated a beautiful prayer of acceptance of God's will for her life:

> Behold the handmaid of the Lord; be it unto me according as Thou will. What a wonderful favor to be chosen as many thousands before, to be the handmaid of the Lord. What return does God expect from me; with what purity of heart and intentions should I make an offering of myself to Him? And

when that offering is made, what a life ought I to lead? I give myself up entirely to Him that He may do with me whatever it pleases Him.[7]

Miss Nightingale displayed the great value she placed on the prayers of others in a letter written to a friend, after learning of the Crimean soldiers' desire to pray for her: "Now I had rather have the men's prayers than a vote of thanks from the House of Commons. And I think there can be no more precious acknowledgement of service done for them."[8] She went on to say, however, that the War Office should not order the men to pray for her but they should be "left to pray willingly," observing: "This is my feeling . . . not because I do not value the prayers of the men but because I value them so much."[9] Finally, Florence Nightingale shared both her Trinitarian theology of prayer and her concept of God's response to prayer in a commentary on the spiritual life:

God does not refuse to answer the longing, devoted spirit which says: 'Speak Lord, for thy loving child heareth.' He hears as the Father; he answers as the Son, and as the Holy Spirit. I could not understand God if He were to speak to me. But the Holy Spirit, the Divine in me, tells me what I am to do . . . this voice is ever beyond and above me, calling me to more and more good.[10]

Nursing publications in the United States began to proliferate in the early twentieth century; following Miss Nightingale's lead, a number of articles of the era dealt with the importance of prayer in the life of a nurse. One example is an article published in *The Public Health Nurse* of June 1923, in which the author asserted that "all who embrace nursing as a life profession must have as a secret source of their ministering contacts" a prayerful relationship with God;[11] and in a 1926 commentary in *The Trained Nurse and Hospital Review*, another author suggested that nurses approach a bedside from a posture of prayer; and added, poetically, that thus: "They meet the waning hopes of the poor bedridden soul with the radiant beams of a morning glimpse of God."[12]

In 1929, the fledgling *American Journal of Nursing* published a poignant epic prayer entitled "Mary's Nurse." The anonymously authored meditation described a "visiting nurse" of the era attending a young mother-to-be on Christmas Eve; the nurse suggested that on this night they should think of another young mother-to-be, Mary, awaiting the birth of her child in a stable in Bethlehem. The nurse observed that Joseph, Mary's husband, had probably sought out a local woman to assist with the birth; as the two made their way to the stable, the meditation continued: "Mary's 'nurse' began to sing of Israel's Messiah and thought to herself 'How glorious 'twould be to nurse into the world the Little Lord ... some day perhaps a woman such as I will have that blessing and that happiness; but I can only bring some comfort now to a poor young girl in a wretched cattle stall.'"[13] The meditation concludes with the visiting nurse imagining Joseph's expression of amazement at the care and generosity of "Mary's nurse" who stayed with the Holy Family throughout the night; when Joseph tried to express his gratitude, the woman replied simply: "It is not hard to nurse the sick for those whose lives are given so. To tend the maimed, the ill, that is a joyous life, a life complete."[14]

The author of a 1937 textbook *The Art and Science of Nursing* advised that the nurse may offer a patient a form of "spiritual therapy" such as "reading from the Bible or saying a prayer";[15] and, a 1939 prayer composed for a school of nursing graduation ceremony, asked that nurses: "in addition to binding broken bodies," be enabled to "heal broken hearts and soothe disquieted minds with the balm obtained from the celestial pharmacy, which strengthens, comforts, cheers and cures."[16]

In her 1945 classic, *The Nurse: Handmaid of the Divine Physician*, Mary Berenice Beck authored a nurse's prayer that read in part: "I am thine own, great Healer, help Thou me, to serve Thy sick in humble charity";[17] a "Night Nurse's Prayer" published in *The Catholic Nurse* in 1954 included the concept of seeing Christ in all of one's patients: "I looked at my patient there in his bed, but I felt I was seeing the thorn-crowned head";[18] and in a 1956 book on moral issues in nursing, an entire chapter is devoted to "The Nurse: A Woman of Prayer." The author asserted: "Because the nurse's vocation is so singularly Christlike, it is imperative that she work though Him, and in Him and with Him. The nurse will find the solution to most of her difficulties, will see her vocation in a new light, through personal contact with Christ. Prayer is that personal contact."[19]

As to contemporary publications in nursing, many "fundamentals" texts include some reference to prayer as a dimension of the nurse's practice; and a recent literature search to identify journal articles focused on the relationship between nursing and prayer revealed 34 publications extant from 1989 to 2000. A search for prayer as a key concept in nursing journal articles under such headings as spiritual care, nursing care, spirituality, nurse-patient relations, and ethics, however, identified 21,319 items.

Finally, in a qualitative study of spirituality and nursing, which I conducted among 66 contemporary nurses, the importance of prayer in the nurse's practice was demonstrated graphically in a theme labeled "Nursing Liturgy." A touching example is an anecdote shared by a pediatric nurse practitioner who described a prayerful "nursing liturgy" carried out prior to the death of an anencephalic newborn:

> The baby, a "preemie," had lived for a couple of weeks, but there were so many congenital anomalies that there was no hope; so the family signed the papers to terminate life support. The parents just couldn't be there, though, so we decided to plan something. It was a very young neonatologist; it was really hard on him, and myself and the Peds ICU head nurse. We came into the NICU (Neonatal Intensive Care Unit) at about 5 A.M. on a Saturday, when there weren't a lot of staff around. We took the baby into a separate little isolation room and discontinued the "vent" and the IVs, all the life support systems. And then we prayed and we sang hymns and we just held her and loved her until she died. It was her special ritual to go to God, and we shared it with her."[20]

PRAYER AND THE CHARISM OF NURSING: DEVOTION TO CARING FOR THE SICK

The concept of charism, especially the charism of nursing, may not be familiar to all nurses. The word *charism*, understood as a special gift from God, has become a well-known term to women religious in recent years. During the past few decades religious communities have been asked to identify and explore from a historical perspective the original charism or gift with which their founder(s) was(were) endowed. It was felt by scholars that this work was critical to the ongoing growth and development of the communities. Such an effort can also be helpful for the contemporary nursing community, especially as related to the meaning of prayer in the life of the practicing nurse.

Prayer

Scripture, in both the Old and the New Testaments, teaches us a great deal about prayer. First, we are instructed that we must pray, and that we must do so with consistency. In the parable of the persistent widow, St. Luke reports that Jesus pointed out to his followers "the necessity for them to pray always without becoming weary" (Luke 18: 1);

and in his first letter to the Thessalonians, St. Paul advised the new Christians to "pray without ceasing," for Paul adds, "In all circumstances ... this is the will of God for you in Christ Jesus" (1 Thessalonians 5: 18).

Jesus taught us how to pray: "When you pray, say: / "Father, hallowed be your name" (Luke 11: 2); and the Lord urged that we be forgiving in prayer, not only in the words of the "Our Father": "we forgive those who trespass against us," but also in such mandates as "Pray for those who mistreat you" (Luke 6: 28); and "Love your enemies, and pray for those who persecute you" (Matthew 5: 44). Jesus also advised his disciples that they should employ prayer in times of crisis: "Pray that you may not undergo the test" (Luke 22: 40). Such advice regarding the power of prayer is supported by the apostle James who wrote to the people of Israel: "Is anyone among you suffering? He should ... pray ... and the prayer of faith will save the sick person" (James 5: 13–15).

In many instances in the New Testament, Jesus is described as modeling the importance of prayer: "He went up on the mountain by himself to pray" (Matthew 14: 23); and on the Mount of Olives: "After withdrawing about a stone's throw from them and kneeling, he prayed saying: 'Father, if you are willing, take this cup away from me; still, not my will but yours be done'" (Luke 22: 41).

And, the fact that the Father hears and answers our prayers is reflected in numerous passages of the Old Testament: "When you call me, when you go to pray to me, I will listen to you" (Jeremiah 29: 12); "And if my people ... humble themselves and pray, and seek my presence ... I will hear them from heaven" (2 Chronicles 7: 14); "The LORD has heard my prayer; / the LORD takes up my plea" (Psalm 6: 10); and similar passages can be found in the New Testament: "Whatever you ask for in prayer with faith, you will receive" (Matthew 21: 22); "Therefore I tell you, all that you ask for in prayer, believe that you will receive it and it shall be yours" (Mark 11: 24); "Ask and it will be given to you; seek and you will find; knock and the door will be opened to you" (Matthew 7: 7).

But what, really, do we mean by the term *prayer* and what does it have to do with the charism of nursing? The word *prayer* has been defined literally as meaning a "petition or request" derived from the "Latin verb *precari*, to entreat or to beg."[21] Christian prayer is broadly understood as a "personal response to the felt presence of God in an effort to intensify that presence" in our lives.[22] Some descriptions of prayer shared by spiritual writers include the following: "a conscious or unconscious revelation of who we are in relationship to God";[23] "a means of giving God thanks and praise and calling upon him for ... daily needs";[24] a time of "learning to listen instead of talk";[25] and, "an affective communication between two persons growing in knowledge, love and intimacy with each other."[26] It is suggested that although "God cannot be co-erced by our desires," this reality does not mean that we should never share them with him in the development of a relationship;[27] a prayerful attitude, however, is characterized by "a readiness to be surprised at every moment by a new call from the Beloved."[28] Ultimately, Brother Roger of Taize advises: "When you understand little of what he expects from you, tell him so. In prayer that is humble, tell him everything, even what you cannot put into words."[29]

Nursing, as a vocation of prayerful ministry to the sick, has survived, along with Christianity, for over 2000 years. We must be doing something right. But what unique spiritual quality is it that characterizes the vocation of nursing? What prayerful whisper of God called forth the nursing of the early Christian deacons and deaconesses who traveled to the homes of the poor to provide care? Who even brought the sick poor into their own homes if need be? What grace so characterized the Crimean mission of Florence Nightingale that she be remembered even today as a "ministering angel" to the sick? And what charism blesses the contemporary nurse who undertakes a ministry of caring in a health care arena fraught with both physical and emotional stressors? What spiritual virtue undergirds such committed nursing practice? The answer, both historically and for the nurse of today, lies in the charism of prayerful devotion: devotion to the sick, devotion to the infirm, devotion to the marginalized, and devotion to the helpless; prayerful devotion to those for whom Jesus taught us to care: the hungry, the thirsty, the stranger, the unclothed, the isolated, and the ill. Nurses' ministry of prayerful devotion lies in our service to God's most fragile and most needy—that is the gift, that is the charism of nursing.

Charism

The term *charism* is derived from the Greek word *charisma* meaning "gift or favor," and it is generally considered "a spiritual capacity resulting from God's grace."[30] Charisms are usually viewed as gifts of the Holy Spirit,[31] to be used for the benefit of others.[32] The exercise of the gifts is motivated by love;[33] and it may be accompanied by "some form of persecution or misunderstanding."[34] St. Paul introduced the concept of charism or religious gift in a number of his letters. In writing to the Hebrews, Paul exhorted the community to faithfulness and assured them that, as an aid to salvation, God distributed "the gifts of the holy Spirit" (Hebrews 2: 4). Paul also acknowledged the pluralism of ministries and gifts in his first letter to the Corinthians: "There are different kinds of spiritual gifts but the same Spirit; there are different forms of service but the same Lord; there are different workings but the same God who produces all of them in everyone" (1 Corinthians 12: 4). It is important to remember that charisms "given to one person can become embodied in a large group … the unique gift of the founder or foundress is given to every member from one generation to the next."[35]

For the contemporary nursing community, examining the concept of devotion to caring for the sick, the spiritual charism of our founder Florence Nightingale and her Christian forebears, can provide important insights both to support a current prayerful nursing practice and to provide direction for future nursing activities.

Devotion

Both the Old Testament and New Testament scriptures give credence to the importance of devotion among peoples. When the Lord mandated Jeremiah the prophet to preach his message to Jerusalem, He said of Israel: "I remember the devotion of your youth, / how you loved me as a bride, / Following me in the desert / in a land unsown. / Sacred to the LORD was Israel" (Jeremiah 2: 2–3); and in Saint Paul's pastoral letter to his coworker Titus, he wrote that certain directives for Christians must be insisted upon; the first of these was "that those who have believed in God be careful to devote themselves to good works" (Titus 3: 8).

The word *devotion* is derived from the Latin *devotio*, and it may be defined as "giving oneself over to someone or something out of permanent conviction."[36] An important characteristic of devotion is prayerful openness to God's call. In his classic work *Introduction to a Devout Life*, Francis De Sales asserted that "Every vocation becomes more agreeable when united with devotion."[37] For the follower of Christ, devotion is identified as "the feeling side of Christian faith," which includes emotional prayer responses to Jesus and to His gospel message.[38] Contemporary spiritual writer Benedict Groeschel describes devotion poetically as "the place where the word of God planted by the Divine sower of the parable takes root in the life and being of the believer."[39]

The previously mentioned characteristics of devotion—the love of God, the unquestioned and total commitment to caring, and the prayerful desire to take on good works, were well exemplified in the first 18 centuries of Christian nursing. Devotion was reflected in the ministries of the deacons and deaconesses, the Roman Matrons, the early and medieval monastic nurses, the military nurses of the Crusades, and the members of the Catholic and Protestant religious nursing communities. Devotion was also a key characteristic of the formal initiation of the profession of nursing, beginning in the Nightingale era of the mid-nineteenth century.

In exploring the life and writings of Florence Nightingale, especially in studying her recorded prayers described earlier, the concept of devotion emerges as the significant gift or charism with which Florence was graced by God. Nightingale not only spoke of the profession of the nurse, or the duty, or the responsibility, although she did use such terms, but she also focused on the spiritual dimension of her calling and of the calling of those nurses who would follow in her footsteps. In one of Nightingale's most frequently cited letters she wrote:

> Nursing is an art; and if it is to be made an art, it requires as exclusive a devotion, as hard a preparation as any painter's or sculptor's work. For what is having to do with dead canvas or cold marble compared with having to do with the living body; the temple of God's spirit?[40]

In a discussion of the ideal characteristics of a nurse, as presented in her classic *Notes on Nursing*, Nightingale asserted: "She must be a religious and devoted woman."[41] And in describing nurses' training at the Kaiserswerth Lutheran Deaconess School, Miss Nightingale expressed her deep admiration for the trainees' commitment: "I have never met with a higher tone, purer devotion, than there."[42]

In commentaries on the life and ministry of Nightingale, one generally finds expressions such as, "She devoted her life to caring for the sick."[43] And, prior to Florence Nightingale's acceptance of her mission to the Crimea, an impassioned appeal to the women of England was published in a London newspaper, which began: "Are there no devoted women among us able and willing to go forth and minister to the sick and suffering soldiers ... in the hospitals at Scutari?"[44] The letter concluded, after applauding France's missioning of sisters to the Crimea: "Must we fall so far below the French in self-sacrifice and devotedness in a work which Christ so signally blesses as done unto Himself, 'I was sick and ye visited me?'"[45] Finally the concept of devotion in nursing as a charism, passed down to her followers by Miss Nightingale, was described in the report of an attending physician of the Scutari Hospitals: "Many devoted females shared [Florence Nightingale's] labors, and greatly to be honored is that company of educated women who with her voluntarily exchanged the comforts and refinements of home for the dangers and privations they were sure to encounter in a military hospital."[46]

It might be summarized that Florence Nightingale's gift of devotion to caring for the sick well fits the definition of charism as a call from God; as service to be used for the benefit of others; as a gift to be passed on to followers; and also as a vocation, frequently accompanied by misunderstanding and opposition. The latter point is reflected in the continual concern about the work of nursing expressed by Miss Nightingale's family who "did not sympathize with her thought of service to the world, but tried to make her see that her place was at home in the ordinary rounds of a woman's life."[47]

The nursing literature immediately following the Nightingale era was replete with references to devotion as a characteristic of the practice of nursing. A 1929 text, *The Ethics and Art of Conduct for Nurses*, included an entire chapter on "The Nurse's Devotion." The "quality of devotedness" the author noted, is a "disposition of heart" that nurses should possess "in a high degree."[48] It is, however, not an easy thing to be "truly devoted," the discussion continued, as devotion requires a complete and unselfish giving of oneself. The characteristics of a devoted nurse were identified as love for the sick, tenderness, generosity, self-forgetfulness, and appreciation for the nobility of the calling. Ultimately, the author concluded, the devoted nurse is prayerfully "consecrated or vowed" to caring for the sick and to relieving suffering.[49]

In our own era, devotion to the nursing profession continues to be reflected in the ongoing clinical practice, research, and writing of nurse practitioners, nurse administrators, nurse educators, and nurse researchers. Prayer and devotion to caring for the sick are as inextricably linked for the twenty-first-century nurse as they were for our nursing forebears. We, as they, face patient and family needs that daily challenge our commitment and our caring. Some days being a nurse may not seem the treasured role we once thought; the many other professions now open to men and women can exert a seductive attraction, especially during stressful times in nursing. But, we as nurses are "vowed"; we are devoted to responding to Christ's call to care for "the least" of our brothers and sisters. And it is this very call, this vocation to nursing, that supports us in the difficult times. It is through prayer and a prayerful response to the call of Jesus that we will receive the grace and the strength to remain faithful to our vow of service.

PRAYER AND CONTEMPORARY NURSING: WHY SHOULD WE PRAY?

One Saturday morning, at an early service on The Catholic University campus, the celebrant chose as the topic for his homily the question: "Why should we pray?" Although I was, admittedly, still a bit drowsy from a late night of writing, my ears immediately perked up. I really need to "get" this, I thought. At the preacher's first comment, however, my heart sank, for he began to quote the great scholar and doctor of the Church, Thomas Aquinas. Aquinas, the celebrant explained, taught that we should pray because of the principle of "secondary causality." "Oh, oh," I lamented to myself, much as I respect and honor the sainted Aquinas, "it's much too early for a philosophical discourse on prayer."

However, and there's usually a "however" in anecdotes such as this, our wise and sensitive homilist was understanding of both the hour and the spiritual needs of the small congregation gathered for worship. He immediately acknowledged that the phrase *secondary causality* sounded pretty intimidating, and he explained that what Aquinas really meant was that God, in His abundant love, allows us, in prayer, to participate as cocreators in his work in the universe. As an example, the preacher cited the concept of rain; because God who created the world knows that the earth needs rain, why should we pray for rain? Not, surely, to attempt to twist God's arm, but rather to cooperate with him in seeking the response to a need.

With this thought in mind, my nurse's imagination was quickly borne away to a past clinical experience. I remembered standing with a mother at the bedside of a 14 year old who had just been diagnosed with a highly malignant anaplastic astrocytoma. I remembered making comments like: "I'll be praying for Michael," and "You are both in my heart and my prayers." Now God certainly knew that Michael was desperately ill. He knew that Michael and his mother needed His comfort and support; and He knew that I, as a nurse, needed His strength and His tenderness to minister to this family. So, why pray for these things?

Suddenly Aquinas's teaching made sense. Yes, God Our Father, in His omnipotence, knows our needs, our desires, and our hopes. But in His great wisdom, He also knows that we desire to participate with Him in the fulfillment of these needs, these desires, and these hopes; when we perceive problems, we long to be part of the solutions. Of course outcomes may not always be as we would wish; that's why we must pray as Jesus prayed: "Father … not my will but yours be done" (Luke 22: 42). But when we pray about the things that are important to us, we recognize the importance of God for us. Whenever we have a personal encounter that involves great joy, great sorrow, or even a profound insight, the first thing most of us do is run to the phone (or perhaps email in this age of communication technology) to share the experience with someone we love. Should it not be the same with the One we love most deeply and who loves us with an everlasting love, the One who is the source of our strength and the center of our lives? Why should we pray? How can we not pray?

PRAYER AND THE PRESENCE OF GOD IN NURSING

It's clear, both from the teaching of scripture and from the understanding of scholars such as Thomas Aquinas, that God desires and welcomes our prayers. We hear, over and over, the messages: "pray always"; "pray without ceasing"; "practice the prayerful presence of God." But how can one accomplish such prayer in the midst of a busy and active lifestyle? How can contemporary nurses manage to "pray always" with the continual mental, emotional, and physical challenges that demand their time and their energies throughout each day? For each nurse the way of living a prayerful life will be different. I believe, however, that we can draw both inspiration and support in the development of our prayer lives from great scholars of prayer such as Thomas Aquinas, Francis De Sales, Jean-Pierre De Caussade and Brother Lawrence of the Resurrection.

In prayer, one focuses on the development of a personal relationship with God. Supportive of this thought are the beautiful words of Francis De Sales, who observed:

> Prayer is opening our understanding to God's brightness and light, and exposing our will to the warmth of His love.... It is a spring of blessings and its waters quench the thirst of the passions of our heart, and wash away our imperfections, and make the plants of our good desires grow green and bear flowers.[50]

In addition to Francis De Sales, two early spiritual theorists of prayer and the practice of the presence of God are the eighteenth-century Jesuit Jean-Pierre De Caussade and seventeenth-century Carmelite Brother Lawrence of the Resurrection.

Pierre De Caussade's small work *Abandonment to Divine Providence* is a classic treatise on the sacrament of the present moment—the prayer of finding God's loving presence in the ordinary moments of our daily lives. There are no moments in our lives which are not holy, for God is present in every moment, De Caussade maintained. "God reveals Himself to us through the most commonplace happenings in a way just as mysterious and just as truly worthy of admiration as in the great occurrences of history and the scriptures."[51]

Brother Lawrence of the Resurrection, who spent the first 15 years of his Carmelite vocation as the community cook, and is thus sometimes referred to as the "saint of the pots and pans," also adhered to a spirituality of practicing the prayerful presence of God in daily activities. Brother Lawrence considered the practice of the presence of God to be the "essence of the spiritual life." "We do not always have to be in church to be with God," he wrote. "Get used to gradually offering God your heart whenever you can."[52] Lawrence, who is described as "the mystic par excellence of the duties of one's state," suggested that while we do need periods of silence before the Lord, we must also take advantage of the many "wasted moments during the day,"[53] and turn our minds and hearts to God wherever we are.

I have a dear friend and colleague who is a community health nursing faculty member and a Sister of Mercy. Sometimes, she drives me crazy; she also teaches me a great deal about the practice of the presence of God, especially when she's driving me crazy. Often I will have something I want to share with her: good news about someone we know, concerns about a school of nursing problem, a thought about our students, and so forth. So, when we get together, I am ready to talk; I am also ready to carry out whatever activities we had planned to engage in: going for a walk, shopping for groceries, or heading off to a meeting. The problem is that as soon as I start to talk, my friend stops moving. I find this very frustrating. I am really not a true "type-A" personality; I need to take time to reenergize both spiritually and physically, but I do like efficiency, that famous American concept. So, I will glare at my friend and grouse: "Why are you stopping? We have to keep moving; we have things to do!" And she, quite calmly, continues to stand still, smiles at me, and replies: "I'm being present to you; I'm listening; I'm giving you my full attention." I generally continue to grump that I do not understand why she can't "be present" to me and walk at the same time but ... I am beginning to get the message. How easy it is to pray and to talk and to write about the importance and the beauty of seeing God, of seeing Jesus, in all those with whom we interact. Yet, if Jesus was really standing beside us and sharing his love or his pain or his concern for the world, would we really want to keep on walking or would we, indeed, want to be as fully present to Him as possible?

Last year I met with a group of 47 practicing nurses who were deeply concerned with the challenge of attempting to incorporate a prayerful practice of the presence of God in their busy workdays. "There is no time for prayer built into present-day nursing schedules" they lamented. And yet, the nurses, all of whom had taken time off for a day of spiritual retreat, admitted to the need for prayer in their lives. We spoke about a number of creative strategies for creating private prayer time; these strategies are discussed later in this book. But the focus of discussion at our meeting was particularly centered on attempting to identify and acknowledge the presence of God within a daily round of nursing activities. Several suggestions highlighted the "sacredness" of the many tasks of caring for the sick. Reflecting briefly on the holy nature of the work either just prior to or immediately following some nursing procedure, someone pointed out that, even while gathering materials to set up an IV or to draw up a medication, nurses can breathe a quick prayer for both themselves and the persons for whom they are about to care. At the conclusion of our discussion, a hospital head nurse shared a prayer strategy that had just come to her as she listened to the ideas of others. She commented:

> I always feel that I don't have time to pray when I'm on duty, but I just thought of something. My office is at the end of a very long hall some distance from the nurses station. I walk that hall many times each day. I just realized that I can begin to use my time of walking down the hall as a time of prayer.

For each of us the creative way of finding time to prayerfully practice the presence of God in our nursing day will be different. But to do so not only will bless and enrich our practice but also will bring a sense of peace and equanimity to our often stressful nursing lives. I believe that such prayerfulness is an absolute necessity if we are to treat our patients with the care and compassion of the gospel message of Jesus, and if we are to approach our patients cloaked in a mantle of compassionate caring.

PRAYER AND THE SURPRISES OF GOD: A NURSE'S VESPERS

Earlier in this chapter, I cited a spiritual writer who suggested that all prayer should be characterized by the readiness to be continually surprised by a new and perhaps different approach from the Lord. This thought reminds me of a favorite passage from Carlo Caretto's commentary on the "Prayer of Abandonment," in which the Little Brother of Jesus admits that God always takes him by surprise. Brother Carlo acknowledged:

> His time has never been mine … When I was waiting for Him under the olive tree, He came under the oak; when I was waiting for Him in Church, He came in the city; when I sought Him in joy, He came in sorrow; when I gave up waiting for Him, I found Him before me, waiting for me![54]

I had a wonderful surprise in prayer this past winter, which I jotted down in my journal; it reflects, I believe, the greatness and the goodness of our God who comes to us, even when we think that events of our lives or of our work may prevent us from coming to Him. The experience provided the unexpected joy of communal prayer; I titled my journal entry "A Nurse's Vespers."

Evening was rapidly approaching on a wintry Sunday afternoon; it was almost time to pray one of my favorite liturgical hours of the day: vespers, or evening prayer. It seemed that my prayer was not to be this night, however, for I was "on duty" in a small makeshift infirmary, created on the ground floor of the Basilica of the National Shrine of the Immaculate Conception, adjacent to The Catholic University campus. The church was, at the time, filled to overflowing with pilgrims, many of whom had traveled from across the country to attend a service celebrating the sacredness of life. I already had one "patient" in our infirmary; a young Sister, very ill with the most recent reincarnation of stomach flu that had been making its rounds of late.

My patient was being tenderly supported by another young Sister, Sister Sarah, who also happened to be a nurse. We did our best to make our Sister patient comfortable, including dimming the lights, in the hope of helping her sleep. As I moved away from the sickbed, I happened to notice that Sister Sarah, who had been assigned to continue in a nursing role while her other Sisters went to pray, had with her a "Divine Office" book that looked identical to my own. As no other patient needs seemed to be immediately on the horizon, I asked the Sister if we two could become a community and pray vespers together; she joyfully agreed.

Sister Sarah and I settled ourselves, prayerfully, on the floor in a corner of the infirmary, using only the soft light from a nearby bathroom to read the psalms and prayers of the Office. I'm not sure if our posture was liturgically correct, but I believe that the Divine Physician, who had, Himself, such tender care and concern for the sick, accepted our evening prayer and blessed our small community. I shall forever treasure the experience of "nursing vespers," which Sister Sarah and I prayed, kneeling on our infirmary floor, as darkness quietly settled over the great basilica dedicated to the Mother of Jesus.

There is a richness of opportunity for prayer in nursing, as in no other profession. Occasionally, we have the gift of time, a brief break, as when we were able to pray our nurse's vespers just described. More often, as noted in the meditation "Contemplative Caregiving," our work must become our prayer. If, however, we live in openness to the surprises of our loving God, a God who is always present and always ready to welcome us to His company, we will indeed be blessed with a deeply fulfilling practice of nursing; a graced ministry of contemplative caregiving to those who are ill and infirm.

A NURSE'S PRAYER FOR DEVOTION

"I remember the devotion of your youth; / how you loved me as a bride, / Following me in the desert / in a land unsown."

Jeremiah 2: 2–3

Oh God, who gifted our profession of nursing with the charism of devotion to caring for the sick, teach me to pray. Bless me with the gift of devout and fervent trust, as you lead my patients into the desert of illness or infirmity. Send your Spirit of wisdom and understanding to guide my mind and my heart as I seek to support the fragile bodies and spirits of those who must walk in a "land unsown." Grace my nursing with an enlivened devotion to You, my Lord and my God, that I may share this precious treasure with all whom you have entrusted to my loving care. Amen.

2 ◈ A Holy Calling: Prayer and Commitment to Nursing

"He told them a parable about the necessity for them to pray always without becoming weary."

Luke 18: 1

THE NURSE'S CALL

The call is so pure; so uncomplicated;
*   "Come follow me."*

O Lord, I want to follow You; it's all
*   I want, really!*
Your voice fills my ears:
*   sometimes, it's as gentle as a soft breeze*
*   whispering through the leaves;*
*   other times, it's as powerful as the*
*   roar of surf in a gale force storm.*

I want to rush after You, panting and out of
*   breath and beg: "I heard Your call to serve*
*   Lord; to care for Your ill and Your infirm.*
*   Wait up, please; I'm coming!"*

That's what my heart aches for, but you
*   know me so well, Lord. There's that*
*   panic that always creeps in.*

21

I feel like Peter skimming the waves;
suddenly I look down and moan: "I
can't do this; I'm not made for
walking on water!"
And, my following You seems to come
to a dead halt.

But You're right there with me, Lord;
tenderly stretching out Your hand.
You give me the courage to try
again, with childlike, tottering
steps, to come to You.

My legs tremble, and my breath comes
in ragged gasps.
The battle has weakened me, but
You're so close now.
I know I can make it.

Finally, I throw myself exhausted
into Your waiting arms,
like a long-distance runner who's
just crossed the finish line.
And the reward is glorious.

Dear Lord,
I heard Your call,
I chose to follow,
I struggled mightily,
You waited patiently,

I'm home!

I have a lovely mid-twentieth-century nursing poster decorating my office wall. The black-and-white ink sketch depicts a 1950s era nurse, elegant in white uniform and cap, with a dark cape billowing out over her slender shoulders. The nurse is pictured with open arms, standing under a life-sized crucifix; the motto on the poster, an advertisement for membership in the National Council of Catholic Nurses, reads "Nursing ... a pathway to sanctity." I love the imagery of the sketch and its message, because they remind me that the nurse's calling is truly a holy one, and that the nurse's calling can indeed become a "pathway to sanctity."[1]

I know that sometimes I am a hopeless idealist; well, quite honestly, most of the time I am a hopeless idealist! But I have learned and continue to learn of so many exquisitely caring attitudes and behaviors among practicing nurses that I believe my idealism is warranted. Recently, a retired nurse walked into my office and challenged me about my writing on spirituality and nursing. I gathered she has not had positive experiences with the current health care system. The nurse commented that my "idealistic" writing about nursing might have been "OK" 50 years ago but she asserted: "You're out of date; it's not like that today!"

That, of course, is one person's opinion. I have the blessed opportunity of continually learning about the meaning of contemporary nursing from students at all levels in my teaching. Some are young baccalaureate nursing students bursting with the excitement of their first clinical experiences; others are seasoned staff nurses or nurse managers, who have returned to school for a graduate degree; the latter have a wealth of experience in clinical practice to share. Most of these students tell the kinds of caregiving stories that bring tears to my eyes and make me incredibly proud of being a nurse. Do they have bad days? Absolutely! I would not be true to the anecdotes the students relate if I were to deny that. But overall, my nursing students, both young and older, are every bit as idealistic as I, and they are every bit as grateful as I for the holy calling, for the pathway to sanctity, which we describe as the profession of nursing.

PRAYER AND A HOLY CALLING

"Be holy, for I, the LORD, your God, am holy."

Leviticus 19: 2

In the Old Testament book of Leviticus, the Lord told Moses to tell the Israelite community to "Be holy," as the Lord, their God, was holy. We, as contemporary nurses, are also called to be holy. But what does "being holy" mean in the twenty-first-century health care arena? How can we really be holy as the Israelites of old in the fast-paced, hi-tech society of today? And is holiness still a value in the nursing profession of the new millennium?

First of all, I suppose, being a nurse researcher, I should explore both conceptual and operational definitions of the word *holy* for nurses; that task would be rather difficult, however, considering the vast diversity of activities within today's nursing profession. A theological definition describes holiness as "the state of being set apart for religious purposes or being consecrated for God."[2] When I think of a person as being holy, I tend to use analogous adjectives such as blessed, spiritual, compassionate, and God-like. Holiness can be described in similar terms for a nurse: compassionate, caring, blessed, spiritual, or God-like in approach to patient care. How a nurse's call to holiness will be lived out, nevertheless, will be significantly different for each caregiver, depending on his or her unique talents and abilities. As the Apostle Peter wrote to the early Christians of Asia Minor:

> As each one has received a gift, use it to serve one another as good stewards of God's varied grace. Whoever preaches, let it be with the words of God; whoever serves, let it be with the strength that God supplies, so that in all things God may be glorified through Jesus Christ.
>
>   1 Peter 4: 10–11

Peter's words seem so beautifully clear and simple: "whoever serves, let it be with God's strength"; that's a lovely thought for nurses, whose calling is about a commitment to serve the sick and the infirm. The problem, for me at least, is how to not lose sight of the fact that my strength comes through Him and in Him and from Him. So often I worry and stew about my ability to accomplish a particular task, totally forgetting that my service is not about my accomplishments but about the work of the One who so lovingly called me to this ministry of caring for the sick. It is only in and through prayer that we can recognize and remember that our strength, our ability to serve the sick, comes from God; and that He who called us to this work will never fail us. I love the concept of the "earthen vessel" as described by Paul in 2 Corinthians 4: 7: "We hold this treasure in earthen vessels, that the surpassing power may be of God and not from us." I value the analogy so much that I wrote an entire chapter on its importance in an earlier book *The Nurse's Calling: A Christian Spirituality of Caring for the Sick.*[3]

Another metaphor that I treasure as a nurse is that of being an "instrument of God," especially as described by spiritual writer Joyce Rupp in her book *May I Have This Dance?* In a beautiful meditation entitled "Instruments of God," the author likens herself to a small hollow flute resting in the hand of God, awaiting the breath of the One who makes melody for the "song-starved world."[4] As a significant portion of my "nursing" these days consists of writing, I like to think of myself also as a small hollow flute, waiting patiently for God to use me to make a "melody" of words. I recognize more and more each day the giftedness of being a hollow reed, whose only purpose is to serve as an instrument of His love for those who are ill and for their caregivers. It is only in prayer, however, that I can become free enough to be used for God's purposes instead of my own, that I can become secure enough to accept personal emptiness, in order that I may be filled with His love.

In a small book entitled *The Call of Silent Love*, a Carthusian novice master reminds us that although God calls all of us to a holy and intimate relationship with Him, He "nevertheless respects our freedom."[5] God will never force us to respond to His call; our response must be, as in any human relationship, one made out of loving and free choice. God is, however, seductive in calling us to holiness. He uses our natural, human desires and attractions to draw us to Himself and to His service. In her comprehensive history, *Florence Nightingale: Mystic, Visionary and Healer*, Barbara Dossey cites a revealing admission of Nightingale's early attraction to nursing

> God has always led me of Himself ... the first idea I can recollect when I was a child was a desire to nurse the sick. My day dreams were all of hospitals and I visited them whenever I could.... I thought God had called me to serve Him in that way."[6]

I wish I could say that I was as holy as Florence Nightingale as a young child but, alas, such is not the case. I was, however, an avid reader of Cherry Ames — *Cherry Ames, Student Nurse*; *Cherry Ames, Graduate Nurse*; *Cherry Ames, Army Nurse*, and so forth. I do not remember all of the titles, but being a somewhat fragile child, I had learned to love reading quite early; it was my way of vicariously enjoying many adventures that my physical strength would not have otherwise permitted. In fact, my mother developed a close relationship with a local bookstore manager, who always saved her a copy of the latest *Cherry Ames* volume, which I would then receive on a special occasion; as a result, I completed my grade school years with a bookcase full of "Cherry's" nursing exploits. And while this collection may not have been a spiritual attraction, Cherry was, in fact, a very moral, ethical, and compassionate nursing model, always putting her patient's needs before her own. Indeed, I believe it was my love of Cherry Ames which led me, as a teen, to begin immersing myself in accounts of the more spiritual vocations to nursing embodied in the lives of such figures as Francis of Assisi, Vincent de Paul, Damien of Molokai, Florence Nightingale, and a host of missionary nurses, whose religious call to caregiving touched the secret desire of my own heart.

PRAYER AND COMMITMENT TO NURSING

"Entrust your works to the LORD, / and your plans will succeed."
Proverbs 16: 3

In 1962, Madeleine Vaillot authored a book on commitment to nursing in which she suggested that the committed nurse "asks to be judged in terms of the values to which she subscribes ... as a nurse."[7] For a committed nurse, the work, Vaillot observed, is a life activity: "It is a form of creative art and the committed nurse may have the urge to do nursing, as the writer must write, the musician must compose and the scientist must do research."[8] A 1982 publication of the National League for Nursing examined the topic in a book entitled *Commitment: A Lost Characteristic*, and it concluded with the recommendation that, among other things, the nursing leadership of the era must seek to "regain commitment as the characteristic that energizes all other components of [nursing] practice."[9] And writing more recently on the concept of commitment in nursing, Verna Benner Carson asserted "commitment requires that nurses make themselves available to others as long as those clients need support."[10] "A committed nurse," Carson adds, "shares in the loneliness, anxiety and suffering experienced by a client and does not pull out of the relationship when it becomes uncomfortable."[11]

In the following pages, the importance of prayerful commitment for present day nurses is explored in terms of the use of the Nightingale Pledge as an oath marking a promotion in status within the educational arena. At my school of nursing, as at many other nursing schools in the country, students commemorate their Commitment to Nursing ceremony by reciting the Nightingale Pledge. In many instances, the wording of the pledge is modified by the students to reflect their contemporary understanding of commitment to the nursing profession. The overall elan, however, of the original nineteenth-century Nightingale Pledge remains intact.

For a number of years, I have enjoyed the prayerful Commitment to Nursing ceremonies that our students have planned. Through those years of watching ceremonies, the outer appearance of the students has changed. While the nursing cap has remained the same, the dress has changed significantly—from the mid-calf, long-sleeved starched white uniform of old, to the shorter, softer white dress of the past few decades, and now, most recently, to the white slacks and jackets that the students find more practical for working in their hi-tech clinical environments. It's true the outward appearance of the nursing students has changed; their inward commitment to the profession, however, is as strong as ever. To document this commitment I decided to explore the original version of the Nightingale Pledge, by conducting a spiritual retrieval of its major concepts in light of contemporary nursing practice.

THE NIGHTINGALE PLEDGE: A SPIRITUAL RETRIEVAL

Chapter 1 included a discussion on the value of seeking to identify a community's original charism or spiritual gift with which God endowed the founder(s). For nursing, the charism of devotion to caring for the sick was described as both the characteristic with which God had gifted Florence Nightingale and the legacy that she passed on to her followers. As noted, many religious communities of men and women are currently seeking to revive and revitalize their founder(s')'s charisms. In a similar vein, some religious groups are also using a theological or spiritual retrieval to conceptualize a contemporary understanding of early virtues embraced by those who founded the communities. One example is the work of Robert Maloney, C.M., Superior General of the Vincentian family, who examined the five virtues identified by Saint Vincent de Paul as important for his followers: simplicity, humility, meekness, mortification, and zeal. Maloney explored the seventeenth-century virtues in light of the "meaning and the forms they might take in the modern world."[12] A similar effort can be undertaken to retrieve the central concepts of the nineteenth-century Nightingale Pledge as meaningful to twenty-first-century members of the nursing profession. This task is both an important and timely exploration because the "Nightingale Pledge," as noted, continues to be used in a variety of forms for present day nursing ceremonies.

The Pledge

A study of nursing history reveals that during the early decades of professional education, schools seeking ethical guidelines for practice developed a variety of oaths and prayers that were recited by the nurses at their graduations.[13] In 1893, however, a committee of nurses chaired by

Lystra Gretter, director of the Farrand School of Nursing at the Harper Hospital in Detroit, wrote a nursing pledge dedicated to Florence Nightingale which became the accepted oath of the profession. The pledge is as follows:

> I solemnly pledge myself before God and in the presence of this assembly to pass my life in purity and to practice my profession faithfully. I will abstain from whatever is deleterious and mischievous, and will not take or knowingly administer any harmful drug. I will do all in my power to maintain and elevate the standard of my profession, and will hold in confidence all personal matters committed to my keeping and all family affairs coming to my knowledge in the practice of my calling. With loyalty will I endeavor to aid the physician in his work, and devote myself to the welfare of those committed to my care.[14]

Historians suggest that one of the advisers to Lystra Gretter's committee was a Harper Hospital physician and thus the Nightingale Pledge contains many similarities to the Hippocratic oath.[15] When one compares the two pledges, certain characteristics emerge in both statements: These characteristics might be said to describe the concepts of "commitment" (Hippocratic oath—an oath before Greek and Roman Deities; Nightingale Pledge—a pledge before God); "community" (Hippocratic oath—recognition of a community of parents, teachers, family members, and disciples as important; Nightingale Pledge—identification of the presence of an assembly during the pledge); "ethics" (Hippocratic oath—abstinence from doing what is deleterious and mischievous, giving deadly medicine and every act of corruption, divulging what should be kept secret; Nightingale Pledge—abstinence from doing what is deleterious and mischievous, taking or administering any harmful drug, divulging personal matters committed to one's keeping); "spirituality" (Hippocratic oath—vow to pass one's life with purity and holiness; Nightingale Pledge—vow to pass one's life in purity and practice the profession faithfully); and altruism (Hippocratic oath—entering houses only for the benefit of the sick; Nightingale Pledge—doing all in one's power to elevate the standards of the profession).

One significant difference in the pledges is that the Hippocratic oath concludes with a prediction that for those who "keep the oath unviolated," they will "enjoy life and practice of the art"; if the oath is violated, however, the reverse will occur. No such statement was included in the briefer Nightingale Pledge.

Several nursing articles have explored the Nightingale Pledge in the last decade, although current commentaries on the oath are few. One important examination of the pledge is that of Judith Calhoun who, while acknowledging certain criticisms of the early message, nevertheless asserts that evidence exists that "threads of the Nightingale Pledge … have been woven into the formal guidelines for the nursing profession of today."[16] Beth McBurney and Tina Filoromo also believe that the pledge has relevance for today's nursing, especially in terms of such virtues as "purity, faithfulness, abstinence, confidence holding, and loyalty."[17] And Teresa Betts-Cobau and Paulette Hoyer contend that the Nightingale Pledge can still be used as an ethical guide for nursing practice.[18]

Spiritual Retrieval of the Nightingale Pledge

The Nightingale Pledge contains key concepts and virtues that might be explored in light of contemporary spirituality in nursing. As noted in Father Robert Maloney's work cited earlier, some of the concepts are not "irrelevant today" even as described in the nineteenth century; however, as also with Rev. Robert Maloney's retrieval effort, in some cases "the language by which [the concepts] are described [is] no longer relevant because of changing times and circumstances."[19] The central concepts that can be derived from the Nightingale Pledge include commitment, community, spirituality, faithfulness, ethics, altruism, confidentiality, loyalty, and devotion to caring for the sick.

Commitment

"I solemnly pledge myself before God."

"This is what the LORD has commanded: When a man makes a vow to the LORD or binds himself under oath to a pledge … he shall not violate his word, but must fulfill exactly the promise he has uttered."
Numbers 30: 3

Commitment is generally understood as making a promise or pledge to do something, and to do it faithfully. The meaning of commitment, especially the concept of vowed or permanent commitment, is something that is discussed a great deal in today's world. Some question the understanding of marital commitment, given the high divorce rate in our society. And yet, commitment remains an ideal that young people continue to find attractive and enticing.

In an exploration of the Nightingale Pledge, on its hundredth anniversary, it was suggested that the words of the oath "imply making commitments."[20] Despite the weakening of commitment in many sectors of today's world, the concept of commitment is attractive to nurses precisely because it incorporates such virtues as fidelity and dedication. In my own school of nursing our students have renamed what used to be called a Capping ceremony, to a Commitment to Nursing ceremony, although "capping" remains the central activity of the service. While the students may never wear their gold-banded nursing caps after the ceremony, they continue to treasure this symbol of their commitment to nursing; students request the religious service of blessing of the caps year after year. As a baccalaureate faculty member who recently assisted at the ceremony put it metaphorically: "The students wear their caps internally; the gold bands are wrapped around their hearts."

I asked one of the recently "capped" students if she would share what the act of making a "commitment to nursing" meant to her as a fledgling nurse. She responded:

> Entering into the health care field in an age when biotechnology and genomics are on the horizon, it has grown increasingly more important to get back to the basics of caring for a client's health. That is, after all what the field is supposed to be about.... Participating in a traditional Commitment to Nursing Capping ceremony afforded me the opportunity to realize this. In her day, Florence Nightingale was a revolutionary, overflowing with ideas that seemed almost too altruistic to be realistic. However, today as we press into the twenty-first century in an entirely different health care delivery system, her values and ideas remain a strong core of the nurse's role. In nursing school we are taught the values of beneficence, veracity, fidelity, and prudence. These virtues are not any less needed today than they were in the Crimea.... Everyday that I look at my cap, sitting on top of my computer, I am reminded of my commitment to a life filled with these values.

Community

"And in the presence of this assembly"

"Sing to the LORD a new song / of praise in the assembly of the faithful."
Psalm 149: 1

A community is "a body of people having common organization or interests."[21] Community, as discussed in Christian Scripture, reflects the greatest commandment of Jesus that one love God first, above all, and that one love one's neighbor as oneself.[22] Nurses are members of a number of communities, especially those related to their individual professional nursing specialties; one of the newest of these specialized communities is that of parish nursing.

Last year I attended a week-long parish nursing course, at the end of which members of the class were commissioned as parish nurses. The course was to prepare us, as licensed RNs, for ministry within our respective faith communities. Twenty-two nurses from a variety of religious traditions, nursing specialty areas, and experiences in parish health ministry were enrolled in the class. The concept, however, that drew all of us to the course and that truly bonded us as a group (we continue to stay in touch by email to this day), was the value we placed upon community, most especially the communities of our personal faith traditions.

Although there are some exceptions, parish nursing is largely a volunteer effort at the present time. I was truly moved during the course by the many touching examples of volunteer nursing ministry shared by the parish nurses. One nurse related how she had organized her church health ministry team to provide respite support for the family of an ICU patient; the family members had been attempting to maintain 24-hour vigils with their loved one. The nurse was able to organize a cadre of volunteers to spend nights with the patient to allow the family some relief; this health ministry was deeply appreciated by both patient and family members — the community of the body of Christ.

Spirituality

"To pass my life in purity"

"Blessed are the clean of heart, / for they will see God."
Matthew 5: 8

The pledge to "pass one's life in purity" reflects a deeply meaningful commitment to a nurse's spirituality. The concept purity of heart "indicates a personal integration, a single-heartedness due to a lack of inner division."[23] As used in the "Beatitudes," purity of heart is described as "singleness of purpose and loyalty toward God" and a conceptualization "more basic than moral purity, for it deals with honesty and integrity in [one's] entire being."[24] "Only this attitude," it is concluded, "leads us to the presence of God."[25]

I love the concept of "purity of heart" because it reflects a spirituality of simplicity and honesty; the idea that all of one's attitudes and behaviors are undergird with integrity. I always worry about the "purity" of my motives; am I truly doing something for the good of others, or is there something in it for me? A friend once reminded me, as I was obsessing over some behavior or other, that our motives are rarely completely pure; this is because of the fragility of our human natures. All we can do is try to embrace those activities and attitudes that are reflective of gospel values and beg the assistance of the Holy Spirit to purify our motives.

I found that I was not unique in my concern about purity of intention when I asked another friend about the concept recently. She admitted:

> When I pray; when I decide to undertake some work, I need to make sure that I'm listening to God and not to myself. I was praying about a trip I was going to take to visit some ill family members and I wondered if I was doing it for them or for my own satisfaction, to make me feel good about myself? But then I thought about how Mary took a trip to visit her cousin Elizabeth when she learned of both their pregnancies, and that's when Jesus was recognized. Jesus is manifested by our presence to each other, so I tried to think of my trip as being in His presence and bringing His presence to my family.

Faithfulness

"And to practice my profession faithfully"

"I give you this command: serve God faithfully and do what is right before him."

Tobit 14: 9

A contemporary text on the fundamentals of nursing explains faithfulness or fidelity for the nurse as referring to an agreement to keep promises: "A commitment to fidelity explains the reluctance to abandon clients even when disagreement arises about a decision a client might make. The standard of fidelity also includes an obligation to follow through with care offered to a client."[26]

I have always thought that the most challenging kind of faithfulness in nursing is the commitment to see a terminally ill client through to the end. We nurses love to see our patients flourish and become physically well under our care; this, however, is not the mission for all of us, especially for those whose nursing vocation is to care for the aged or the terminally ill. I asked a hospice nurse, Margaret, whose vocation for 20 years was the care of dying cancer patients, what had kept her faithful to her calling. She observed that it was a spiritual philosophy of nursing which had enabled her to do the work for so long; the idea of "not deserting the Body of Christ." Margaret added: "I think I received the gift of a contemplative vision of going beyond caring for the patient's physical body to caring for the wounded Jesus. I tried to do the nursing to the best of my ability, but it was not really me who did it but the Christ within me. I also tried to treat each patient as I would treat Christ." Finally, Margaret concluded: "I had fun too. You've got to have a sense of humor; God does. I really enjoyed the patients and the families and the volunteers I worked with."

Kathleen, another long-time nursing colleague, also shared a lovely thought on the concept of practicing her profession faithfully. She explained that her early nursing education had taken place in a hospital that was described in its original charter as "a chapel with wards attached." Kathleen admitted: "I don't wear the cap anymore; it gets in the way of my stethoscope. I don't wear the pin either, because I fear I might lose it from the lab coat that is now my uniform. But those words have guided my actions as faithfully as is humanly possible and I am grateful."

Ethics

"I will abstain from whatever is deleterious and mischievous, and will not take or knowingly administer any harmful drug"

"Abstain from every kind of evil."

1 Thessalonians 3: 22

Ethics is defined in a current nursing text as a "systematic inquiry into principles of right and wrong conduct, of virtue and vice, and of good and evil as they relate to conduct."[27] It is also noted that the term *professional ethics* usually relates to attitudes and behaviors incorporated into a "code of professional conduct such as nursing codes of ethics."[28] Judith Calhoun, in her commentary on the Nightingale Pledge, asserts that the "threads" of the oath are in fact incorporated into our contemporary ethical codes of nursing.[29]

Nursing ethics is a difficult concept to address from a clinical perspective, because the principle of "doing no harm" is universally adhered to by most practicing nurses; case study material would primarily involve negative exceptions, which, thank God, are few. Perhaps what should be applauded and imitated in contemporary nursing are those activities that not only are ethical but that also go far beyond the usual or expected professional responsibilities.

An example that comes to mind is the commitment and support provided to families of those who have died while in a nurse's care. Very often oncology nurses, hospice nurses, ICU nurses, AIDS nurses, and nurses from a variety of other specialties attend funerals or memorial services to honor deceased patients and to provide a compassionate health care presence for the families. This kind of informal nursing activity is long cherished in the hearts and minds of bereaved family members.

Altruism

"I will do all in my power to maintain and elevate the standard of my profession"

"This is why I have raised you up, to show my power through you that my name may be proclaimed throughout all the earth."
                                                            Romans 9: 17

Quite honestly, I was having some difficulty coming up with a concept that seemed to capture the Nightingale Pledge's mandate to "maintain and elevate the standards of the profession." As a sort of "working concept" I labeled the thought altruism. Great was my surprise when I discovered that two newly published nursing textbooks identified altruism as one of the recommended professional values for nurses. The 2001 edition of Potter and Perry, defines altruism as "concern for the welfare of others.... [The nurse] gives full attention to the client when giving care; assists other personnel in providing care when they are unable to do so; expresses concern about social trends and issues that have implications for health care."[30] The fourth edition of Taylor, Lillis and LeMone, also 2001, suggests, in a similar vein, that "Altruism is a concern for the welfare and the well-being of others. In professional practice, altruism is reflected by the nurse's concern for the welfare of patients, other nurses, and other health care providers."[31] Some professional behaviors identified by the authors include understanding other cultures, serving as patient advocate, risk-taking for patients and coworkers, and mentoring.[32] These two definitions of altruism in nursing do indeed reflect the concept of elevating the standards of professional nursing.

There are many examples of altruism among twenty-first-century nurses. Perhaps because of my own long academic career, my thoughts are immediately directed to the activities of nurses who, for some at great personal sacrifice, continue to further their education to elevate nursing standards and behaviors. This may mean returning to school for an advanced degree, or it may mean faithfully attending professional conferences and workshops to remain current in one's specialty area. All of these activities can be costly both financially and in terms of time and energy.

I asked a doctoral candidate at my school of nursing, much of whose career has been in nursing practice, why she had embarked on doctoral education. She explained:

> So that I can teach others the things I am learning. Jesus teaches us to go to the poor and the sick. Hopefully through my teaching I can share my love of the Gospel; I can share my care for those who are poor and sick. I'm doing a doctoral dissertation about homelessness so that the homeless can teach me about spirituality in their lives. I can talk about the subject, write about it, teach students. I can help students see that people without homes are people of God, just like us. I will have more to teach the students with this degree.

Confidentiality

"And will hold in confidence all personal matters committed to my keeping and all family affairs coming to my knowledge in the practice of my calling"

"He who betrays a secret cannot be trusted, / he will never find an intimate friend. / Cherish your friend, keep faith with him; / but if you betray his confidence, follow him not; / For as an enemy might kill a man, / you have killed your neighbor's friendship."

Sirach 27: 16–18

Most contemporary nursing texts include some comment about the patient's right to be assured of confidentiality, especially in terms of formal health records: "Patients have a moral and legal right to expect that the information contained in the patient health record will be kept private."[33] Perhaps the more delicate issue in terms of confidentiality, however, is the privacy with which a nurse must hold confidences shared verbally by a patient or family member. Have we not all, on at least one occasion, experienced a "change of shift" report in which a nurse, perhaps in a burst of excitement, divulged some private information about a patient or family member? Unfortunately, most of us, and I have to admit to heading the list, enjoy hearing some fascinating tidbit of heretofore unknown information about someone we know. Nevertheless, we need to continually put ourselves in the place of the patient whose trust, even if unwittingly, might be violated.

An oncology nurse told me of a patient care situation in which she felt that holding a verbal confidence was very difficult. A dying patient had told her something that he did not want his family to know. This information could, however, have made the family members, some of whom were distanced from the patient, view his life and past behavior in a much more positive light. The nurse would have liked to reveal the information but that was not the patient's wish. She commented: "All I could do was try to be a gentle intermediary when the family was there and try to facilitate their good-byes."

Loyalty

"With loyalty will I endeavor to aid the physician in his work"

"Of kindness and judgment I will sing: to you, O LORD, I will sing praise."

Psalm 101: 1

This statement is perhaps the most controversial in the Nightingale Pledge for some contemporary nurses. Not the loyalty part, which I will address first, but the final phrase of providing "aid (to) the physician"; it does not, however, need to be so.

The topic "conflicting loyalties and obligations" of the nurse is a subtopic in the Kozier, Erb, Berman, and Burke fundamentals text of 2000. Judith Wilkinson, the author of the chapter on values, ethics, and advocacy, admits that "Because of their unique position in the health care system, nurses [may] experience conflicts among their loyalties and obligations to clients, families, physicians, employing institutions and licensing bodies."[34] It is asserted, however, that "According to the nursing code of ethics, the nurse's first loyalty is to the client."[35] To discuss such conflicting loyalties and professional responsibilities in depth is beyond the scope of this book. Suffice it to say that while the nursing guidelines are clear, the concrete patient, family, physician, or institutional interactions within which the nurse may find him or herself may not be so. Prayer to the Holy Spirit of Wisdom and Truth and the wise guidance of a trusted spiritual advisor can provide the best direction for resolving such clinical conflicts.

The concept of "aiding" the physician has been identified as problematic for some nurses in the recent past because of the desire for autonomy in professional nursing practice; that desire, however, I would argue, has now been accomplished in large measure. In most of the clinical situations in which I have worked, and in the anecdotes I hear from practicing nurses, contemporary physicians welcome the input and advice of nurses as fully participating members of the health care team. Are there exceptions? Of course. To deny this would be naive, but I do believe that instances in which nurses are not respected or not valued by the physicians with whom they work are few and far between in today's health care system.

One practicing nurse I discussed this concept with put it this way:

> Well, we all work together. I think you need to define the word *aid*. Do I ever "aid" the physician in the process of making a patient well? Yes. As a nursing supervisor my goal is quality patient care. I make sure the patients are comfortable, the staff have what they need, even housekeeping; they all interact with the patient. By doing this I am "aiding" the physician in his work because I am facilitating the healing of the patient. By doing good nursing I am aiding the physician in his work of healing. This idea of aiding the physician is not a problem for me; we all ask for help and aid each other. Think about the scripture when we say to the Lord: "O God come to my assistance; O Lord make haste to help me."

Devotion to Caring for the Sick

"And devote myself to the welfare of those committed to my care"

*"Those who have believed in God (should) be careful to devote them-
selves to good works; these are excellent and beneficial to others."*

Titus 3: 8

The concept of devotion to caring for the sick, as the charism of
Florence Nightingale, and ultimately the charism of the modern nursing
profession she founded, is explored in Chapter 1. The elements of devotion highlighted here are the characteristics of commitment and hard
work, which support and undergird the art and the practice of devotion
to caring for those who are ill. As Nightingale noted: "Nursing ... requires
as exclusive a devotion, as hard a preparation as any painter's or sculp-
tor's work";[36] devotion in nursing, our founder asserted, is not easily
come by.

Perhaps the best example of a nurse's devotion to caring for the sick
I can think of is that of a missionary nurse who is a dear friend and mentor of mine. Ellen was nursing in a developing country at the time the
HIV/AIDS pandemic began to be recognized worldwide; in the late 1980s
and early 1990s. While there was, in the United States, an explosion of
information about the virus and related illness syndromes during the
early years of the pandemic, HIV information was very slow in becoming
public in Ellen's country. Long after U.S. nurses were exposed to comprehensive data describing methods of transmission, nurses with whom
Ellen worked were still terrified to enter the room of a person with HIV
infection. Thus, my friend embraced the commitment and the hard work
of gathering and disseminating as much current information about HIV
and AIDS as she could find. She provided "hands-on" care for patients
personally to model her lack of fear before hospital nurses; she spoke at
nursing and medical meetings; she wrote about the illness. She even returned home to the States to gather the latest HIV information to bring
back to her adopted country in order to continue the work of caregiving
and education; her ministry continues today. In her continual and abiding
devotion to the welfare of the HIV infected persons who have been committed to her care, Ellen truly exemplifies both the mandate of the
Nightingale Pledge and the charism of our profession.

Overall, the clinical attitudes and activities just described document
that, while terminology may differ, the basic concepts of the Nightingale

Pledge continue to be respected and embraced in the experiences of contemporary practicing nurses. Earlier in this chapter, I posed several questions related to how a nurse might live out a holy calling of commitment to serve the sick in today's hi-tech health care arena. Virtually all of the nurses with whom I have discussed this topic, admit that their ability to be faithful to their vocation of committed service and to the concepts identified in the Nightingale Pledge is through a prayerful approach to their nursing.

PRAYER AND THE NIGHTINGALE PLEDGE

When he was in prison, incarcerated because of his faith, Saint Paul wrote to the early Colossian Christians, encouraging them to live a holy life. Paul admonished the new Christians: "Put on then, as God's chosen ones, holy and beloved, heartfelt compassion, kindness, humility, gentleness, and patience, bearing with one another and forgiving one another" (Colossians 3: 12). I often wonder, am I holy in my nursing? Do I really try to live out the virtues encompassed by my vocation to serve the ill and the infirm? I am encouraged by the words of spiritual writers such as William Rademacher who reminds us that "After Christ's resurrection, all of creation, including 'everyday things' is holy again.... Time is holy and filled with encounters with the holy for those believers who have eyes to see and ears to hear. The present moment is indeed a sacrament."[37]

This work of being holy, of embracing the Nightingale Pledge is not any easy task. That, I believe would be admitted by all of the nurses described earlier; that's why the idea of a prayerful approach to living out one's vocation is critical to so many practicing nurses. I began this book by quoting a Benedictine prioress who had commented that living without prayer "doesn't work"; I added my thought that nursing without prayer doesn't work. I believe that the latter maxim becomes a living reality when one considers the virtues in the Nightingale Pledge. Nursing characteristics such as commitment, faithfulness, altruism, loyalty, and devotion are not easily come by for we ordinary humans. They are gifts and graces we must seek from the Lord in humble and heartfelt prayer.

Later chapters in this book explore such topics for nurses as methods of prayer, strategies for incorporating prayer in work and leisure, and discernment of God's will in prayer. As I was thinking of the kind of prayer that might be derived from the Nightingale Pledge it struck me that, related to the nurse's calling, a psalm of reverence for the sacredness of all human life would be an appropriate theme for meditation.

A NURSE'S PSALM OF REVERENCE FOR LIFE

Oh, Lord our God, I praise you
for the gift of life.
When I see a newborn infant, the
work of your hands;
A mother's love, the tenderness
of your care.

Who are we that you bless us
with the sacredness of life;
that you create us to serve
each other with caring
and compassion.

For the chronically ill, who find in
their infirmities, the power
of your strength,
I praise you O Lord.

For the mentally challenged, who engage
their lives with bravery and
gentleness,
I praise you O Lord.

For the physically handicapped, who clothe
their disabilities with
dignity and grace,
I praise you O Lord.

For sick children, who embrace their
illnesses with courage and
simplicity,
I praise you O Lord.

For frail elders, who boldly refuse
to "go gently" into the
night,
I praise you O Lord.

For loving families, who tenderly
support disabled
members,
I praise you O Lord.

For loyal friends, who faithfully
attend to the needs of ill
comrades,
I praise you O Lord.

For the blessing,
and the holiness
and the giftedness
of all human life,
I praise and thank you
O Lord.

A NURSE'S PRAYER FOR FAITHFULNESS

"We know that all things work for good for those who love God, who
are called according to His purpose."

Romans 8: 28

O God, who called me to this holy ministry, keep me faithful to my
vocation. Help me to make of my nursing, a prayer of commitment
and caring. Let me recognize every sickroom as a tabernacle where
You dwell. Direct my work that it will become a prayer of reverence
and respect for the sacredness of human life. Bless me, always, with
a grateful heart, that I may be ever mindful of the precious gift of
serving You in the ill and the infirm. Amen.

3 ▨ Openness to the Spirit: Prayer and Becoming a Vessel

"With all prayer and supplication, pray at every opportunity in the Spirit."

Ephesians 6: 18

THE NURSE: GOD'S VESSEL

Vessels hold all kinds of blessed things:

> *food and drink to nourish the body;*
> *candles and perfumes to nourish the spirit;*
> *the light of Christ to nourish the soul.*

Vessels are treasured when empty;
> *they can be filled.*
Vessels are precious when full;
> *they can be emptied.*
Vessels may break;
> *they can be mended,*
> > *stronger, often, for the*
> > *sealing of the breach.*

Nurses are called to be God's vessels:

> *to be empty, awaiting the fullness*
> *of His love;*
> *to be full, awaiting the emptiness*
> *of self-giving;*

43

to be broken, in the service of
the sick;
to be stronger, for the healing
of the wound.

It was a lovely late Autumn evening and the majestic one-hundred-year-old chapel on my university campus was filled to overflowing with young people. Students, from a variety of disciplines, had put their busy lives on hold to attend an hour of praise and worship of the Lord. I arrived to find that two of my favorite nursing students had saved a "seat" for me between them on the crowded chapel floor. I love to attend praise and worship with the young ones; their devotion and prayerfulness touches my heart and inspires my own desire for contemplative prayer. I also find these evenings of worship to be a wonderful opportunity to listen to the gentle whisperings of the Holy Spirit. That evening, as I sat amidst the students, listening to them lovingly sing the words "Break my heart Lord," I knew beyond all doubt that the Spirit of God was blessedly among us. As the old hymn put it: "There's a sweet, sweet spirit in this place, and I know that it's the Spirit of the Lord."

The hours of worship are held later in the evening, to accommodate students' schedules, and I must confess that sometimes, after a long day in the school of nursing, I arrive pretty worn out. I often wonder if I have enough energy left to praise the Lord. It seems, however, that it is precisely on those evenings, when I am most tired, that the Lord lifts me up, that He erases my fatigue and sends His Spirit to sustain my flagging energy. I may come to praise and worship feeling like an empty vessel; I leave feeling the fullness of His love. Another of God's surprises!

And isn't it often like this with us as nurses? We spend a busy day pouring out the love and the caring with which the Lord has graced our fragile earthen vessels, and when we finally get around to spending time with Him, we feel too tired to pray. But this is exactly the time we most need to listen, to open our weary hearts and minds that the Spirit of the Lord may fill us again with His strength and His peace.

NURSING PRAYER AND OPENNESS TO THE SPIRIT

"As the hind longs for the running water, / so my soul longs for you, O God."

Psalm 42: 2

Becoming a compassionate and contemplative caregiver does not happen all at once. In a way, the process occurs almost as Margery Williams described "becoming real" in her wonderful allegory *The Velveteen Rabbit*: "It doesn't happen all at once.... You become. It takes a long time."[1]

So, how do we as nurses begin the process of becoming contemplative caregivers? And isn't the word contemplative usually reserved for monks and nuns, living isolated from the world in silent and solemn monasteries and convents? Is it really possible for us to be contemplative in the midst of our ever-changing and ever-challenging contemporary health care system? I would argue that, despite these concerns, most nurses do desire to live a contemplative caregiving life; to serve, in the perception of the great Teresa of Avila, as the hands and the feet and the eyes of the Lord, in caring for their patients. And this is precisely where the gift of learning to listen to the whisperings of the Holy Spirit in our lives comes in.

I have loved and leaned on the Holy Spirit for a very long time it seems. As a young Sister, wearing a religious habit, I was allowed to attach one personal medal to the 15-decade rosary hanging from my belt. I chose a rather large silver medal imprinted with the image of a dove and the words *Veni Creator Spiritus* (Come Holy Spirit). Now, some 35 years later and no longer wearing the habit, I still carry that medal on my key ring; it is a constant reminder of the Holy Spirit's treasured presence in my life.

But who, in fact, is this enigmatic Spirit, this third person of the Blessed Trinity, whom we tend to sometimes refer to as the "Breath of God"? One of the best parts about working on a book like this is that I get lots of "on the job" training, not only in practicing my topics such as prayer and openness to the Spirit, but also in studying about them. So, I have had a chance to explore again some theological understandings of the Holy Spirit upon whom I so depend.

When we look at the New Testament, we find that Jesus told us that the Spirit was to be our advocate, our teacher, and our guide: "The Advocate, the holy Spirit that the Father will send in my name—he will teach you everything and remind you of all that [I] told you" (John 14: 26). A Bible dictionary describes the Holy Spirit as "The mysterious power or presence of God in nature or with individuals and communities, inspiring or empowering them with qualities they would not otherwise possess ... the Spirit of God."[2] A theological definition of the Holy Spirit associates the Spirit with the Hebrew word *ruah* meaning breath or wind; and

identifies the theology of the Holy Spirit as "pneumatology."[3] (Paren-
thetically, I have to confess here that when I first encountered the word
pneumatology early on in my theology studies, I, the self-appointed class
nurse, generated much mirth among my seminarian classmates by in-
sisting that the term sounded more like a chronic lung disease than a
theological concept.) Finally, a dictionary of spirituality asserts that Christian life is "led in the power and under the guidance of the Holy Spirit."[4]
By definition, the Holy Spirit in Christian theology is "the third person of
the Trinity, distinct from but consubstantial, coequal and coeternal with
the Father and the Son, and in the fullest sense, God."[5]

Having said all that, it would surely seem appropriate that we listen
to the guidance of the Holy Spirit in prayer. In fact, Saint Paul taught that
because "we do not know how to pray as we ought," the Spirit comes to
assist us in our weakness and Himself "intercedes" for us with a love and
a care that is beyond words (Romans 8: 26–27); that is, the Holy Spirit
prays for us as well as guiding us in prayer. In a spiritual conference given
to monastics, it was pointed out that the Holy Spirit does not reside pas-
sively in us but is rather an active presence, in that He is "Love, life [and]
light because [He] is God."[6]

But how does one begin the prayerful activity of being open, of
listening to the voice of the Holy Spirit in one's life? In the Introduction to
this book, I suggested that prayer is very much like nursing; it is a practice discipline. In fact, there can be a kind of science as well as an art to
prayer. One may read books on prayer, use the scriptures or other spiritual reading to initiate prayerful meditation, and place oneself in a
prayerful atmosphere to avoid distraction and promote an open mind and
heart. Ultimately, however, just as in nursing practice, the person who desires to pray must simply plunge into the activity with a willing heart and
a loving spirit. This is not always easy; a later chapter deals with such
issues as dryness and distraction in our prayer life. Nevertheless, try we
must, if we are serious about being open to the Spirit of God and to
listening to His voice in our lives.

LISTENING IN NURSING: THE WHISPERING OF THE
HOLY SPIRIT

As nurses, we learn to listen and to listen well. We listen to administrators' goals for our health care facilities; we listen to physician's
directives; and most importantly, we listen to the needs and concerns of
our patients and their families to determine the best plans of care for those

we serve. But, as I noted earlier, sometimes after a long day of listening to our patients, we find ourselves too fatigued, distracted or overwhelmed with worries to be still and listen to the Lord.

I just picked up a newly published book whose title *Armchair Mystic: Easing Into Contemplative Prayer* intrigued me. The author, Mark Thibodeaux, S.J., identifies four stages of prayer: "talking at God" (I do that a lot!); "talking to God" (I'm trying to do that more!); "Listening to God" (I really want to do that!); and "Being with God" (The ultimate desire of my heart!).[7] I think many of us are pretty good at talking to and with God; it's the listening that is the tough one. Thibodeaux notes that moving from those first two stages to listening to God is an "important step" in one's prayer life. When we reach this stage in prayer, he asserts, the focus shifts from one's "own agenda" to "God's agenda." The hard part about listening is that because we cannot actually hear God's voice with our ears, we "simply have to trust that God is present in [our] prayer. That is part of the surrendering that prayer demands."[8]

For me, attempts at listening to the Lord occasionally come easily, but more often, they are difficult. I daydream; I worry; I think about what work I have to do next; I think about what work I have just completed and did not do as well as I think I should have; I think about my needs; I think about my friends' needs and on and on. When I realize that I am not praying at all during a supposed time of prayer, I get embarrassed before God. This embarrassment, of course, is very silly because God knows me so well, so much better than I know myself, and He really does love me anyway. But maybe it's good to be a little embarrassed; that way, at least I can begin to think about the fact that I should be listening to the One I call the source of my strength and the center of my life, instead of acting as if I were all alone in my small universe of needs and concerns.

Psychologist and spiritual writer Benedict Groeschel urges us to listen to God with both our minds and our hearts, and to continually relate the occurrences of the external world, perceived by our senses, to our interior prayer life.[9] Perhaps, one morning, I have meditated on the scripture passage "whatever you did for one of these least brothers of mine, you did for me" (Matthew 25: 40). In my prayer, and my listening to Jesus' words in scripture, I am filled with the desire to take care of each patient I serve, as I would care for Jesus. Then when I arrive at work, I learn that a very fragile homeless person has been admitted to our unit; he has multiple physical and emotional deficits that will make developing and implementing a nursing care plan very difficult. This is a perfect opportunity to listen, both to the voice of the Spirit in my prayer and to the voice of the Spirit in my nursing. If I care for this patient with the love and the respect and the gentleness with which I would treat Jesus, I will, as Benedict Groeschel advises, have listened and prayed with both my mind and my heart.

DISCERNMENT IN NURSING: SEEKING GOD'S WILL

"If you are willing to listen, you will learn; / if you give heed, you will be wise."

Sirach 6: 33

"Here I am [Lord] ... speak, for your servant is listening."

1 Samuel 3: 4–10

"Mary ... sat beside the Lord at his feet listening to him speak.... [Jesus said]: 'Mary has chosen the better part and it will not be taken from her.'"

Luke 10: 38, 42.

Sirach, a sage in early Jerusalem; the ancient author of the Book of Samuel; and Jesus, as described by Saint Luke in his gospel, all tell us that if we "listen," we will learn God's will; we will discern his desire for our lives. In the last quarter century it seems that the word *discernment* has become the "in" terminology for the process of seeking to identify God's calling for an individual. A number of books have been written about spiritual discernment; religious groups conduct discernment retreats for potential applicants; and many faith communities organize discernment workshops for their members. I am currently coleader of a Women's Discernment Group sponsored by the Campus Ministry department at my university.

In the "old days," we simply prayed, and sometimes sought advice from a spiritual mentor, to help us hear God's call; today we discern. Is there a difference? Perhaps in how we go about the process, though not in terms of the overall aim of the effort. In his fine book *Listening to the Music of the Spirit*, Jesuit David Lonsdale asserts that spiritual discernment involves active and conscious engagement with God on the part of the discerner. "Discernment," he believes, means:

ultimately ... placing ourselves as unreservedly as possible in God's hands; asking God to shape our lives through our decisions and thus allowing God to bring to fulfillment the creative work that God has already begun in us.... Discernment involves making choices within a setting of prayer, of a continuing dialogue with God.[10]

And in *The Discerning Heart*, spiritual director Maureen Conroy suggests that discernment is both an art and a skill: an art in that "we pay attention to the mystery and the beauty of God's personal love for us," and a skill, as "we sift through our reactions to God's outpourings of love."[11] Thomas Green adds that discernment can only be learned "by doing"; this he points out is the "relevance of prayer to discernment."[12]

Personally, I agree with the explanations of discernment offered by these scholars of spirituality much wiser than I. A problem that I often encounter in my own experiences of discernment, however, and that I touched on earlier, is the worry, even in prayer, about whether I am really discerning God's will or simply reinforcing my own. Some years ago, I went very excitedly to a friend of mine to share the news of a recently "discerned" decision to undertake a new nursing ministry. I expected a reaction of enthusiasm and excitement which would match my own. Instead I came away from our meeting feeling as if a bucket of at best cool, and at worst very cold, water had been poured over my inflamed spirit; my friend's immediate response was "I'm not sure if you are hearing God's voice or your own."

This was a relevant question, surely, and one to indeed ponder in any serious effort at discernment. After much prayer, I did in fact, modify my plan, although I still undertook a dimension of the ministry to which I had felt called. My discernment resulted not only from prayer and my friend's advice but also from seeking the guidance of a spiritual director and doing some fairly extensive reading in the area of discernment. The latter two activities taught me that, in spiritual matters brought to the Lord in prayer, usually the deepest desire of one's own heart is also the desire of God for that individual. I found that position wonderfully validated in an admission by Gerald May who reported that when he needs a "specific answer for a hard question," he often gets into "a spoken dialogue with God." He asks the questions and God answers, but then, of course, he wonders, as do I, if the answer is really from God or from his own ego. May concluded: "So I ask God, 'God is that really You or me?' The response comes back, 'Yes.'"[13] I like Gerald May.

Might a discerner still be left unclear after a period of discernment is completed? Sometimes. But I believe that, as in the case of my own nursing ministry discernment, continued openness in prayer, continued listening for the quiet, gentle voice of the Holy Spirit, ultimately provides the stimulus and the practical means necessary to respond to the call that is the desire of one's heart of hearts.

THE USE OF SCRIPTURE FOR PRAYER IN NURSING

Spiritual writer Peter Kreeft advises that "praying by reading the gospels prayerfully and 'listeningly' is one of the very best ways to pray."[14] In a later chapter of this book, the specific Scripture-based prayer of *Lectio Divina* is discussed; here the concept of beginning to learn to use Scripture as an adjunct to prayer is introduced. Although it might seem a given that listening to or meditatively reading the word of God would be helpful to prayer, I believe the topic bears some exploring. For myself, as perhaps for a number of other nurses, interest in Scripture may not have been a life-long experience.

My love of Scripture is, in fact, the product of a later-in-life experience of studying the Word of God. To explain that I need to share a little personal history which I do not think will be surprising to the more mature, translated older, Roman Catholic reader. I grew up in a devout Irish Catholic home. The house was filled with devotional articles particular to our faith. There was a kitchen Madonna over the stove, a "Last Supper" in the dining room, and a painting of "Jesus, the Good Shepherd" in the foyer. There were rosaries, medals, and prayer books in abundance, as well as all manner of blessed oils and containers of "holy water" in our home. My father prayed daily from a small prayerbook whose pages were thin and yellowed from use; and often when I came in from school, I would find my mother on her knees praying the rosary while waiting for the family to assemble for dinner.

Yet, in the midst of this wealth of religious devotion, I cannot remember any of us reading the Scriptures. In fairness to my parents, I need to admit that I have a vague memory of a large family Bible that would be retrieved from a closet shelf to record key events such as births, deaths, and first Holy Communions. After each entry, however, the Bible was tucked away again to be reserved in pristine condition for future such occasions. In that era of Catholicism, reading of the Word was primarily carried out within the context of worship services such as the Holy Sacrifice of the Mass.

Although as an adult I experimented with the monastic practice of *Lectio Divina* (reading and meditating on Scripture), it was not until my theology studies a few years ago that I truly came to appreciate the beauty and the power of the Word. I fell in love with the Scriptures. I purchased Bibles of every size and translation. Although I have since given many away, I still keep a Bible in my office, a Bible in my room, and a small Bible in the glove compartment of my car, just in case I get held up in a line of traffic.

But how does one begin the exercise of praying with Scripture? I remember one of the supervising ministers in my hospital chaplaincy program warning us that although we should surely encourage Scripture reading among our patients, we should not advise a neophyte to begin studying Scripture without any guidance. There is a multiplicity of spiritual books to assist in the exercise of praying with Scripture such as *Pray the Bible* by Page Zyromski;[15] and many relevant chapters in books on prayer, for example "Listening at Prayer with the Written Word";[16] "Pondering the Word";[17] and "Contemplating Scripture."[18] There are also Bible dictionaries and commentaries that help explain the meaning of more obscure Scripture passages, as well as providing the history of the holy word; one simple and useful example is the *Collegeville Series on Books of the Bible.*[19]

For many of us, it may be easier to begin with the New Testament — with Scriptures familiar from our worship services: the four gospels; the Acts of the Apostles; and the letters of Jesus' disciples: Paul, James, Peter, John, and Jude. Or we may wish to pick an Old Testament passage with which we also have some familiarity such as the story of Jeremiah and the Potter's Wheel (Jeremiah 18: 1–6), or the prophet Isaiah's promise that those who hope in the Lord will "soar as with eagle's wings" (Isaiah 40: 31). The Psalms are also a wonderful guide to prayer as they are the prayers that Jesus prayed. Each psalm has a unique theme that might be relevant to a particular prayer concern such as praise, thanksgiving, trust; prayer in time of illness; prayer in distress; confidence in God; prayer for help against unjust enemies; prayer for protection; and prayer for faithfulness. Finally, to identify those Scripture passages that may be helpful in prayer, a concordance or dictionary of Scripture references is a wonderful guide to finding one's way around the books of the Bible.

In a chapter of *The Hungry Heart* entitled "What Is the Use of Praying with Scriptures?" Pierre Wolff suggests that a simple answer might be to use Jesus' own words: "Blessed ... are those who hear the word of God and obey it" (Luke 11: 28).[20] Wolff goes on, however, to enumerate a number of other ways in which scripture can help us pray. Some of these include "A Mirror," specific stories to which we as individuals can relate such as the parable of Mary and Martha; the experience of elder "brothers and sisters," as Jeremiah and Judith of the Old Testament; and messages from God revealed through God's interactions with His people.[21]

In terms of the history of our own profession, it has been well documented that Florence Nightingale was an avid reader of the Bible; she wrote many annotations on the Scriptures in which she personally identified with the struggles and experiences of biblical figures.[22] This kind of personal acknowledgment of God's word is a wonderful way to integrate scripture into our prayer lives. I recently admired an older Bible belonging to one of my colleagues at a parish nursing conference. At first she was surprised at my admiration and envy; her Bible was, she admitted, beginning to "fall apart." But what had touched me was the very fact of how worn and well used the treasured Bible appeared; there were handwritten marginal notes on virtually every page for, as with Florence Nightingale, the nurse had personally identified with many Scripture passages. I found myself not feeling terribly proud of my own relatively new looking Bible, which had been in my possession many years less than that of my friend.

PRAYER AND BECOMING A VESSEL: THE SANCTUARY LAMP

"Jesus spoke to them again, saying 'I am the light of the world. Whoever follows me will not walk in darkness but will have the light of life.'"

John 8: 12

At the beginning of this chapter, I mentioned the majestic one-hundred-year-old campus chapel where I love to pray. A special joy is that the chapel happens to be housed in the residence hall where I live. The tabernacle, containing the presence of the Lord, is situated at the front of the church, atop a high stone altar designed in the Gothic style of the Middle Ages. On the altar, next to the tabernacle, is a simple, yet elegant, sanctuary lamp holding a lighted candle; the symbol of Jesus' sacramental presence in the church. It may seem strange to admit, but I love it when the candle flame extinguishes in my presence. I have discovered where the backup stash of sanctuary lamp candles is hidden and have adopted, as my informal sacristan responsibility, the relighting of the lamp with a new candle.

I treasure this task, for I experience an incredible sense of awe and reverence when I climb the steps of the high altar, kneel humbly before the presence of Jesus in the tabernacle, and place the softly glowing candle in its beautiful sanctuary lamp. I feel as if I am, in a way, proclaiming to all who will enter the chapel: "This is Jesus. He is indeed the light of the world." Mother Teresa used to love to say that we do not need to do great things, only "small things with great love." For me taking on this small sacristan activity is a simple yet powerful way of doing a very ordinary thing with great love; it is a way of practicing to become, in all things, His vessel.

In the meditation at the beginning of this chapter, I described the nurse as "God's vessel." I think the true beauty of a vessel is that the vessel, in itself, is of no real use; it's kind of like the lovely story of the "Giving Tree." A vessel is only important for that which it holds: a vessel containing a beautiful bouquet of spring flowers to decorate a room; a vessel holding a fragrantly scented candle to soothe the spirit; a vessel holding sweet, fresh milk to nourish the body. Once these vessels are empty, they are put aside on a shelf until called again into service to provide for the pleasure or comfort of others.

As I looked at the nursing literature, both old and new, I found that I am not alone in seeking to acknowledge nurses as God's vessels. Writing in 1945, Mary Berenice Beck, in her prayer entitled "The Uniform," asked of the Lord: "Hide Thou my raiment from all sight but thine, beneath the nurse's dress that now is mine";[23] and in a *Journal of Christian Nursing* article published 54 years later, the author writing about "work as worship" reported: "I fervently asked that my identity would come from being in Christ and ... not from any other role."[24] It especially moved me, as I searched the older nursing literature, to also discover that often articles dealing with spirituality and nursing were published under anonymous authorship; the nurse authors seeing themselves, perhaps, as hidden vessels or instruments to be used by the Lord, as needed, to represent His care and compassion for those in need.

I believe that the only path to becoming a vessel is through God's grace; a beautiful vessel is created and refined only by a long and sometimes challenging process of prayer and service. I do, however, trust with all my heart, that we as nurses are called to be God's vessels, and that is indeed the greatest gift of our vocation:

to be empty, awaiting the fullness
of His love;
to be full, awaiting the emptiness
of self-giving;
to be broken, in the service of
the sick;
to be stronger, for the healing
of the wound."

A NURSE'S PRAYER FOR THE GIFTS OF THE SPIRIT

"The Advocate, the holy Spirit, that the Father will send ... he will teach you everything, and remind you of all that [I] (Jesus) have told you."

John 14: 26

Come, Holy Spirit, and grace me with the openness to hear your voice and to do your will. Bless my nursing with Your sacred gifts:

Grant me wisdom in making clinical assessments; understanding in listening to patients' needs; knowledge for carrying out therapeutic interventions; right judgment in identifying illness symptoms; courage in implementing aggressive therapies; reverence in supporting patient and family concerns; and wonder and awe at seeing Your presence in each person for whom I care. Teach me, dear Holy Spirit, to be to all I serve, a vessel of your love. Amen.

4 🖾 A Sacred Covenant: Prayer and the Nurse-Patient Relationship

"When you call me, when you go to pray to me, I will listen to you."
Jeremiah 29: 12

A CRACKED VESSEL: THE NURSE'S COVENANT

O God of love and covenant,
  I want so much to be like You;
    to be gentle,
      to be kind,
        to be faithful;
    to be a small and perfect
      earthen vessel,
  ever available for Your use
    in my nursing.

But, Dear Lord, I'm so unlike You.
  So often I allow myself
    to be ungentle,
      to be unkind,
        to be unfaithful;
    to be a small and imperfect
      earthen vessel,
      disfigured by cracks
        on every side.

And my heart breaks, O Lord of my
life, for I fear You could
never choose such an
unworthy receptacle
to become a
source of
Your love
and
Your light
for
the ill and the infirm.

But, You know that this earthen
vessel is made of clay, Dear
Lord; You who tenderly
asked the prophet Jeremiah:
"Can I not do with you
as the potter?"

Yes, Lord, God of love and covenant:
You may indeed do with me as
the potter.
Remold this scarred and damaged
vessel; remake it into the
crucible which You would
have it become.

Let Your light shine forth from this
fragile earthen pot, Dear Lord,
so that the sick who draw from its
contents may know the
glorious power of
Your covenant
and
Your care.

I have prayed a lot about being an earthen vessel; the beautiful analogy that Paul so eloquently shared with the early Christians always brings me a sense of deep joy: "We hold this treasure in earthen vessels, that the surpassing power may be of God and not from us" (2 Corinthians 4: 7). It means that we, fragile as we are, have the magnificent privilege of holding this precious treasure: the "light (shining) out of the darkness"; the light that "has shone in our hearts to bring to light the knowledge of the glory of God on the face of Jesus Christ" (2 Corinthians 4: 6). I pray about this message for I feel such an unworthy vessel. It's easy, especially when I am caught up in my daily nursing education activities, to forget about being a vessel, to forget about the gift of being a treasure bearer.

When I pray about the vessel analogy, I often think of myself as a "cracked vessel"; as a small earthenware pot with lots of scars and gouges garnered over the years, a vessel perhaps not so pretty to look at. When I shared that image with a group of my nursing students one day, a nurse practitioner responded: "Well, with all those cracks just think how much better Christ's light will be able to shine through your earthen vessel."[1] Students are such wonderful teachers.

Because of the fragile human condition, because of our universal earthen vesselness, prayer is critically important to those of us who, as nurses, are ministers to the ill and the infirm. Thus, I struggled mightily with how to begin discussing the varied dimensions of prayer for a nurse. Initially, I thought that the relevance of prayer to the nurse-patient relationship should come first as it is for our patients that we, as nurses, exist. As I prayed about my approach, however, I came to the conclusion that because we stand on the shoulders of those who have gone before us, some exploration of the history of prayer in nursing, of the relationship of the nurse's calling to prayer, and of a nurse's openness to God's will in prayer must precede a more pragmatic clinical discussion. Now, though, it is time to get to the heart of the matter—to the heart of the role of prayer in the life of the practicing nurse and to the nurse-patient relationship. And, in using the label "practicing nurse," I am including not only clinical nurses who physically stand at the bedside of those who are ill, but also those of us who stand figuratively as practitioners, yet whose primary professional nursing role may be that of administrator, manager, teacher, or researcher.

NURSING: A SACRED COVENANT

"I have made a covenant with my chosen one."

Psalm 89: 4

In two previous books on spirituality and nursing, I described the nurse-patient relationship as a "sacred covenant."[2] As I had pondered the concept of God's covenant with His people during my Old Testament studies (e.g., Genesis 9: 8; Genesis 12: 9), I began to think about how a nurse's relationship to his or her patient models a covenantal relationship. There are mutual obligations and responsibilities that must be undertaken, bonds of loyalty, fidelity, and commitment to the covenant.[3]

References to God's covenant with His people abound in both Old and New Testament Scripture. In Genesis, the Lord is reported as telling Noah and his family "I am now establishing my covenant with you and your descendants after you" (9: 9); in Psalm 25, a prayer for guidance, the psalmist asserts "All the paths of the LORD are kindness and constancy / toward those who keep his covenant and his decrees" (v. 10); and, after the birth of John the Baptist, his father Zechariah praised the LORD saying: "Blessed be the LORD, the God of Israel ... / [he has shown] mercy to our fathers ... / mindful of his holy covenant" (Luke 1: 68, 72).

A covenant is defined in the theological literature as "a binding agreement between two parties";[4] it is also described as "one of the bible's most important and pervasive means of describing the relationship between God and the community of faith."[5] A number of theological/spiritual articles deal with the concept of a person's covenant with the Lord. During the past two decades, the nursing literature also has begun to reflect an interest in the covenantal relationship, as a model for nurse-patient interactions. A classic article is that written by Mary Cooper entitled "Covenantal Relationships: Grounding for the Nursing Ethic." The author takes the position that the nurse-patient relationship is indeed a covenantal relationship. "It is a relationship grounded in the moral principle of fidelity and characterized by mutuality, reciprocity, and responsiveness on the part of both the patient and the nurse"; Cooper believes that such covenantal relationships undergird the nursing ethic and promote healing for both nurse and patient.[6]

Two recent nursing journal editorials also support the concept of the nurse-patient covenant, especially in light of the country's contemporary health care system. A 1997 editorial in the *Massachusetts Nurse* acknowledged the difficulties of practicing nursing in a managed-care health care system and encouraged nurses to keep their "covenant to care";[7] and a 1998 editorial in the *Archives of Psychiatric Nursing* entitled "The Nurse-Patient Covenant and the Imperative to Care," also urged practicing nurses to maintain their "professional covenant" with their patients.[8]

Distinguished Quaker spiritual writer Richard Foster urges the importance of "covenant prayer," which he describes as a call to a "God-intoxicated" life. Foster asserts that "God rushes to us at the first hint of our openness" and places in our hearts "an insatiable God-hunger to respond to his covenant of love."[9] But how do we bring our response to this sacred covenant of God's love into our nursing practice? First, we must establish our own personal relationship with the Lord.

PRAYER AND THE NURSE'S RELATIONSHIP WITH GOD

Simon Tugwell, in his book *Prayer: Living with God*, explained that "prayer is not another part for us to act; another skill for us to master; another subject to study for an examination; it is a relationship with God."[10] Richard Foster observes that there may be times in prayer when we are "invaded to the depths by an overwhelming experience of the love of God."[11] Jesuit William Barry gives an example of such an occurrence in relating an anecdote of walking by the sea and being filled with "a feeling of great well-being and a strong desire for ... the 'All,' for union" with God; this, he reports, made him "very happy."[12]

A few years ago, when I was participating in an interview to intern for a hospital chaplaincy program, my prospective supervisor asked if I had ever had an occasion of prayer such as those just described. I rather hesitantly admitted that, yes, there had been an experience: "I'd never dare call it mystical," I added, "but it was surely profound." Why would you be afraid to call the experience mystical, my interviewer questioned? "Well," I hurried on, "I certainly didn't see any visions or hear voices" (I could envision my chaplaincy internship rapidly heading down the drain); but "my spirit was deeply moved. In fact," I asserted, "it's the reason I'm here today, seeking to expand my nursing ministry."

About three years earlier, I had visited, for the first time in many years, a religious setting that was very special to me; the place was the community Motherhouse, now referred to as a "Center," where I had lived as a young Sister. The reason for my visit was ostensibly to participate in a weekend of spiritual retreat and of renewing old friendships. I had a strange feeling, one of those intuitive things you just cannot quite get ahold of, that the Lord wanted me to make this particular pilgrimage. There were a number of legitimate excuses not to go, but as I told a friend: "I have the feeling that I have a date with God."

I arrived at the Motherhouse on a Friday evening, the day before the scheduled activities were to begin. Although the Sisters on the planning committee invited me to an impromptu evening get-together for early arrivals, I begged off with the excuse that I wanted to spend a little quiet time with the Lord.

I visited the Motherhouse chapel and several other favorite spots on the grounds. Although the land and gardens surrounding the Center are usually quite lovely, the season was late winter; the trees still bore barren branches and new life among the plants and flowers had not yet begun to blossom forth. To make things a little more dreary, an all-day March drizzle had permeated the entire East Coast. It was so damp and chilly out that I found myself turning up my trenchcoat collar and shivering as I walked the Motherhouse grounds. Actually, I was about to return to my room for a hot shower and an early-to-bed when I remembered that I had not visited one of my very special places, the Cloister Chapel. As it was getting late, I did not want to ring the entry bell, disturbing a small group of cloistered Sisters, but, I reasoned, I could walk up the path to where the chapel stood and say a prayer, and then I would turn in.

It's really quite difficult to describe what happened next, and perhaps that's why I have never written about it before. As I began walking the path to the Cloister, I abruptly stopped still in my tracks; I was suddenly filled with an overwhelming sense of joy and of love. The thoughts that permeated my heart and my spirit were "This is where your treasure is; this is where your heart is, in His love. Nothing else is important." And in that brief moment, I knew that I had come home; home to that place where Jesus was the center of my life. And I knew also that I would spend the rest of my days, and the rest of my career as a nurse, seeking to live, as Richard Foster so poignantly put it, a "God-intoxicated" life. Because truly, nothing else really does matter.

Do I live this intensely loving relationship with God, each moment, in my life as a Sister and in my work as a nurse academician? I wish it were so, but my human frailty allows me to become so caught up in the cares and worries of the day that I often forget who I really am, and who God really is in my life. Despite my many failures to love and to serve, however, that experience will always be with me, remembered as vividly as if it had occurred yesterday; it is the undergirding theme of my desired relationship with God. When I become anxious and distressed about how little I seem to love, how little I try to live the depth of my covenant relationship with the Lord, I remember a wonderful anecdote related by Benedictine Joan Chittister and it gives me courage. As the story goes, a visitor to a monastery asked one of the older monks "What do you do in the monastery?" And the monastic replied: "Well we fall and we get up, and we fall and we get up, and we fall and we get up."[13] The falling, I think, is not a problem; the secret is never failing to get up.

Each nurse's relationship with God will be, as all relationships, unique and personal. How we interact with the Lord in prayer may differ vastly, but the most important thing is that we do pray, and pray faithfully. For it is only in prayer that we can truly live the sacred covenant of caring that so blesses the nurse-patient relationship.

PRAYER AND THE NURSE-PATIENT RELATIONSHIP

Contemporary nursing texts describe the nurse-patient relationship variously as a nurse-client relationship, a therapeutic relationship, a helping relationship, and an interpersonal relationship. All of these concepts describe the interactional relationships between nurses and those for whom they care. The nurse-patient relationship is considered to be "central to every nursing activity";[14] a "growth-facilitating process" for the client;[15] and "aimed at realizing mutually determined goals" of both patients and nurses.[16] It is suggested that in a nurse-patient relationship, the nurse brings all of her knowledge, skill, and values to the interaction. If, then, prayer is a value for the individual nurse, it is expected that he or she will incorporate some dimension of prayer into the nurse-patient interaction. Depending upon the openness of the relationship, and the particular religious beliefs and traditions of the participants, a nurse may not deem it appropriate to pray with a patient; the nurse may, however, choose to pray for the patient or about his or her nurse-patient interactions. There are a multiplicity of ways such prayers may be approached.

Most scholars of prayer believe that "there are no infallible techniques to prayer that will lead to a deeper relationship with God; there is only a longing of the heart to follow where prayer leads."[17] While accepting this basic posture for approaching prayer, I still believe, however, that prayer, like nursing, has a dimension of being a "practice discipline." This understanding is supported by the vision of Sister Corita Clark who, while acknowledging that we are taught to pray by the Holy Spirit, nevertheless admits that there are things we can do to "facilitate the spirit of prayerfulness" by embracing such aids to prayer as: silence, solitude, discipline, and awareness of the Lord.[18]

The desert fathers and mothers of old taught of the value of silence and solitude, the importance of going away to an isolated place to pray. In a more practical vein, Saint Francis De Sales advised, "Remember to retire at various times into the deserts of your own heart."[19] For most of us a physical "desert retreat," although something I would highly recommend, will not be a frequent experience. While we may not be able to travel to a real desert, many of us can, however, periodically spend a week, a few days, or even a few hours of quiet prayer and reflection at a retreat center or house of prayer. Sometimes, though, because of the demands of work, family, and community activities, even a formally scheduled time of retreat is difficult to achieve. Does that mean that we must give up the idea of silent and solitary prayer? Absolutely not. And that is what Francis De Sales, who so understood the demands of ordinary life, wanted to remind us. For it is, in fact, through small disciplined times of solitude and silence, even if briefly interspersed among our daily activities, that our spirits are fed and our souls nourished with the food of God's love and His caring. It is these brief moments of reflecting on the awareness of God's presence in our lives that will inform and bless our nursing and allow us to truly become contemplative caregivers.

But how, in reality, is such prayerful practice of the presence of God incorporated into the nurse-patient relationship? I believe that prayer is the heart of the caring relationship established between nurses and their patients; and the burden of establishing a prayerful bonding is on us as nurses. I once heard a scholar of prayer advise that one should pray when healthy, for it can be very difficult to pray when one is experiencing a debilitating illness. Our patients may not have the strength, or the powers of concentration, to stay focused on prayer for very long; we can, however, witness for them a prayerful practice of the presence of God in our gentle and tender caring for their bodies and their spirits.

I am reminded of a caregiving situation of many years ago that taught me much about the importance of prayer in my relationship with patients. I was assigned to care for Rachel, a young mother with terminal cancer; being in her early twenties, Rachel was not much older than I was at the time. This was, also, I need to point out, in the days when we did not have either the powerful chemotherapeutic agents or the effective pain and nausea control therapies of today. A new dimension of the caregiving experience for me was the fact that, although I was working in a Catholic hospital, my patient was from an Orthodox Jewish tradition. I prayed a lot about my nursing relationship with Rachel. I grew to love her deeply for her kindness and her strength and her courage; she was also a true woman of prayer. I frequently told Rachel that I was praying for her, and she responded with gratitude. It did not matter that my prayers were Catholic rather than Jewish; we both treasured the act of placing our needs in the hands of the Lord of our lives, and this became our special connection. The unique bond of a prayerful relationship erased any boundaries that our different ethnic or religious affiliations might have raised.

I still remember one evening, when Rachel was nearing death, that my patient, now also my friend, told me how she would love to have a real kosher corned-beef sandwich; that of course was only a fantasy because her stomach had been viciously invaded by the metastatic carcinoma that had begun in one breast. As we laughed about how such a treat might not be a very good idea, I confessed that I, the product of a dyed-in-the-wool Irish-Catholic family, had never even tasted such a delicacy. The next evening Rachel's young husband, whose heart was breaking over the illness of the wife he adored, arrived bearing my supper from a local delicatessen: a magnificent kosher corned-beef sandwich. I cried a lot as I tried to enjoy this special gift of love, the fruit of a prayerful nurse-patient relationship with this beautiful and courageous young mother and wife, who was soon to be with her God.

FINDING TIME FOR PRAYER IN NURSING: AN "ORATORY OF THE HEART"

Brother Lawrence of the Resurrection, the earlier identified "saint of the pots and pans," asserted: "It is not necessary for being with God to be always at church. We may make an oratory of our heart wherein to retire from time to time to converse with him."[20] Jean-Pierre De Caussade, the master of abandonment to Divine Providence, taught that: "the duties of each moment are shadows which hide the action of the Divine will."[21] And, soldier saint Ignatius Loyola believed that for those who "want to love and serve God in all things" love should be manifest "more by deeds than by words."[22] Other scholars of prayer suggest that we may incorporate prayer into our busy days by such activities as thinking of God as we are walking about or working at some manual task; praying the "Jesus Prayer," using a brief formula such as "Come Lord Jesus" or simply repeating the name of Jesus; and meditating on the holiness of ordinary tasks, especially those involving the care of a brother or sister in need. Nursing practice, in its many and varied dimensions, surely lends itself to the latter kind of prayerful meditation.

As noted in Chapter 1, the authors and editors of a number of contemporary clinical nursing journal articles identify prayer as a dimension of the nurse's role. The cover design for a spring 2000 issue of *The Clinical Journal of Oncology Nursing* promoted an article on spiritual care, highlighting the concepts of healing, medicine, faith, and prayer.[23] Prayer has been identified as included in the role of the holistic nurse;[24] the school nurse;[25] the ICU nurse;[26] oncology, hospice, and parish nurses;[27] and as a general nursing intervention in a variety of other nursing areas.[28] It is, thus, a given that most nurses, or at least many nurses, consider prayer to be an important dimension of their practice. But then we must return to the topic of finding time for prayer, or for creating an "oratory of the heart," in the midst of our busy schedules.

Spiritual writer Pierre Wolff takes up the topic boldly by entitling a chapter on prayer "How Can I Pray When I Am Too Busy?" Wolff responds by describing the married relationship of two friends; it is a "love story," he says, "as prayer is." In the anecdote, Wolff explains how his friends, although busy with work, children, and community activities, find time to nurture their love for each other. They may have just a minute to say "I love you," or a longer time to spend being together, but constantly sharing their care for each other has become a way of life. It made me smile to read some of Wolff's descriptions of the couple's expressions of care such as "Love you, running!"[29] because sometimes I do the same thing with the Lord. I feel kind of silly, but I also feel like I am staying connected. For example, the other evening I went to the chapel in my residence hall to pray. I was, however, nursing a nasty ear infection, and as soon as I knelt down, I realized that somebody had left the majority of windows open during the day; the chapel was very cold and damp. So, I said to the Lord: "I think I'd better not stay here too long; love You, back soon!"

Another strategy that helps me to remember to "pray always," or to try, as Pierre Wolff suggests, to pray even when I am too busy, is to decorate my living and work spaces with spiritual/religious pictures and thoughts. I have mentioned one of these already, my NCCN poster reminding me that nursing can be a "pathway to sanctity." I also have a beautifully carved wooden crucifix on my office wall, given to me many years ago when I entered religious life; and a print of Domenico Fetti's 1622 oil painting entitled *The Veil of Veronica*, which one of my students brought me from the National Gallery of Art. Above my computer is a special favorite, a framed print of Jean-Francois Millet's magnificently prayerful painting *The Angelus*. The mid-nineteenth-century scene depicts two young farmers, standing heads bent in prayer, in a potato field, as the sun sets in the background. In the distance one can perceive the faint outline of a village church steeple, its bells tolling the evening Angelus to call the community to prayer. Looking at this print always makes me want to stop for a moment and pray, wishing that I might be united with these young peasant farmers who had interrupted their field work to pay homage to their Lord.

I realize that I am blessed in having an office where I can keep reminders of prayer. I do, however, live in a very small dorm room at my university. And although the living space is limited, I try there also to keep a few miniature prayerful images. It helps me to have a small framed print of the Madonna and Child and a Prayer to the Holy Spirit on my desk. These kinds of prayer aids are within most people's budgets, can be chosen according to individual spiritual/religious taste, and may draw one's thoughts to brief moments of prayer during the busy days when we truly seem to "have no time to pray."

The attraction to particular religious symbols or religious art will be different, of course, for each of us. But being surrounded by things that touch the heart and lift the spirit can be very helpful in supporting an ongoing prayer life. There will, in the trajectory of one's developing spiritual life, always be times of distraction and dryness; these are dealt with in a later chapter. Nevertheless, using natural God-given gifts such as religious art or uplifting spiritual meditations may strengthen one's commitment to prayer and inspire perseverance in attempting the seemingly impossible gospel mandate to "pray always."

PRAYER AND NURSING PRACTICE: A NURSE'S SABBATH

There are many ways to approach a discussion of prayer and nursing practice, because our workplaces are so varied in the contemporary profession. We are hospital nurses, clinic nurses, nurse practitioners in offices, home care nurses, long-term care nurses, parish nurses, military nurses, and nurses employed in other disciplines and settings too numerous to name. Within these arenas, we are nurse clinicians, nurse administrators, nurse managers, nurse educators, and nurse researchers. We are told in the gospel of Jesus that when we care for the sick, we care for Him, that, in fact, our nursing becomes our prayer. But are all of our nursing tasks of equal value? Do they all constitute living the gospel message of Jesus?

A tale from the desert fathers reminds us that a great variety of good works are blessed by the Lord: "For scripture says that Abraham was hospitable and God was with him. And David was humble and God was with him. And Elias loved solitary prayer and God was with him. So, do whatever you see your soul desires according to God."[30] I love that desert fathers' story, because it reminds me that there are many options to serving the Lord for us as nurses; there are many prayerful ministries of caring for the sick which reflect the gospel message: "I was ill and you visited me." In order, however, to be sensitive to prayer, to the need for prayer in the nursing workplace, we also need to have some private time, some "Sabbath time," to be alone to talk with and to listen to the Lord.

The Sabbath is an important day for many major religious traditions; it is a time of rest and relaxation from the workweek, but most importantly, it is a time of prayer, both individual prayer and community prayer. Most Christian denominations hold communal worship services each Sunday (or Saturday, for some). For Roman Catholics, Sunday or Saturday evening Mass is a mandate of the Church; and for many Jewish communities, Sabbath temple worship is expected each week. Because of the importance of the concept, theologian Abraham Heschel wrote a book, now a classic, entitled *The Sabbath, Its Meaning for Modern Man*. In the book theologian Heschel wrote: "Six days a week we wrestle with the world, wringing profit from the earth; on the Sabbath we especially care for the seed of eternity planted in the soul. The world has our hands, but our soul belongs to Someone Else."[31]

The problem, of course, is that nurses often do not have a Sabbath in terms of a particular day of the week. Our Sabbath may consist of 8 to 12 hours staffing an intensive care unit or an emergency room; we may be out in the community doing home care visits to those unable to travel because of illness or disability; or we might even be physically at our respective churches, yet involved in such activities as blood-pressure screening or health counseling in the role of parish or church nurse. It's true that such nursing ministries can themselves constitute prayerful efforts, yet we truly do need some time and place of Sabbath, apart, for our personal communion with the Lord. How can this be accomplished?

The Sabbath spirituality of Abraham Heschel holds that on the Sabbath we must attempt to avoid the tyranny of things and "try to become attuned to holiness in time."[32] I would suggest that because we nurses may not always have one full Sabbath day during a week, although when possible that would surely be desirable, we may, instead, try to create several small Sabbath experiences within the seven-day period. During those mini-Sabbath times, we can embrace Heschel's concept of becoming "attuned to holiness." Our Sabbath experiences might take place on a quiet Sunday evening, a free Wednesday morning, or a Friday afternoon, before a family dinner or weekend activities take over our lives. Communal worship services may need to be worked around our nursing schedules but this is always possible. Nurses are consummate improvisors; one thing I am certain of is that if a nurse sets out to make something work, it will work.

What I am suggesting is surely not new; it's the way a number of nurses have created their Sabbath times for many years. In the early days of nursing education, or "training" as we called it back then, students, and sometimes graduate nurses, had only one free afternoon a week and that rarely fell on a Saturday or a Sunday. And yet, as our history documents, nurses throughout the centuries have included a prayerful spirituality as a significant dimension of their nursing practice. The challenge for us, as contemporary nurses, is to continue in the footsteps of those who have gone before us and to continue our commitment to a prayerful and sacred covenant of caring as we carry out our nurse-patient interactions in the sophisticated health care milieu of the twenty-first century.

A NURSE'S PRAYER OF COVENANT AND CARING

"I have made a Covenant with my chosen one."
Psalm 89: 4

O God of covenant and caring, teach me to reverence relationships. Let me honor the gifts you give so abundantly in the sacred relationships of Your Blessed Trinity. May I revere the blessings of Divine Fatherhood in the person of You, Yahweh, my God; may I treasure the joy of Divine Brotherhood in the person of Jesus; and may I rejoice in the support of Divine Friendship in the person of the Holy Spirit. Help me to model my nursing relationships to reflect Your image and likeness. May I bring to my interactions with those I serve: the parental care of You, God my Father; the passionate love of Your Son, my Lord Jesus; and the inspired wisdom of Your Holy Spirit of understanding and truth. Amen.

5 🔲 Compassionate Caregiving: Prayer and Embracing Patients' Needs

"Have no anxiety at all, but in everything by prayer and petition, with thanksgiving, make your requests known to God."
Philippians 4: 6

A SACRED PLACE OF SILENCE IN NURSING

There's so much noise, Dear Lord,
    and so much pain;
        and
so very many wounds needing to
    be healed.
Some days it almost overwhelms
    me.

I yearn to be alone with You
    in a place of silence;
I long to fill my ears with the
    whisperings of Your Holy
        Spirit;
I ache to immerse my heart in
    the compassion of
        Your care.

In the midst of my hectic nursing
days, I thirst for an oasis of
solitude, where my
parched soul can
be quenched with
the living waters
of Your love.
I hunger for a banquet of peace
where my starving spirit can
be nourished with the
tender quiet of
Your love.

Free me, O Lord, from the prison
of my frantic activity;
extricate me from the
binds of my overcrowded
schedule; liberate me
from the constraint
of my anxious
thoughts.

Lead me, gently, O Lord, to that
sacred place of silence,
hidden in the recesses of
the human heart.
For, it is there that You dwell,
Dear Lord;
it is there that you enfold
my vulnerability with
Your strength;
it is there that You
teach me
the true art
of
compassionate caring.

Mentor my nursing, O Lord, in the
quietness
of
Your love.

"LITTLE MAGGIE"

Her baptismal name was Margaret Anne, but "Little Maggie" was the family's pet name for one of our favorite pediatric patients. She was only 5 years old, but "Little Maggie" had already suffered enough for several lifetimes. Maggie had beautiful blue eyes and a headful of golden curls. Lying on her side in the hospital crib, she appeared the picture of healthy, happy childhood, until one caught sight of the huge invasive tumor disfiguring the tiny face. Olfactory meningioma was the diagnosis; inoperable! Maggie's parents kept a "before" picture on a table near the door. They wanted her nurses and visitors to "see Maggie as they saw her" they told us.

Jody, a pediatric nurse practitioner, entered the room to start a nutritional IV; she had never cared for Maggie before. The parents watched guardedly for their new nurse's reaction: surprise, shock, horror, or even worse. Maggie looked frightened.

Jody approached the hospital crib smiling warmly; she slowly lowered the safety rail and bent over close to Maggie's face. "I'm your nurse today, Maggie," she said, gently ruffling Maggie's curls. "I hope we can be friends." The caring, the compassion, and the tenderness in Jody's eyes were enough. Maggie smiled brightly; her parents shoulders sagged in quiet relief — another parable of nursing compassion.

COMPASSION AND PRAYER IN NURSING

When I began to explore the concept of compassion as related to prayer in nursing, I discovered that the term *compassion* is often used interchangeably with such words as *pity, empathy, sympathy,* and *caring.* This is particularly true in Scripture. My concordance listed a number of New Testament references identified with the term *compassion,* i.e., Matthew 14: 14, Jesus' "compassion" for the crowd; Matthew 20: 29-34, "The Healing of Two Blind Men," during which Jesus was moved with "compassion"; and Matthew 15: 32, "The Feeding of the Four Thousand," when Jesus said, "My heart is moved with 'compassion.' When, however, I looked up these references in the biblical translation I was using at the time, the word *pity* was substituted for *compassion* in each passage.

One reference, interestingly, in which the word *compassion* is actually used in the passage title is that in which Jesus is described as caring for the sick: "The Compassion of Jesus. Jesus went around to all the towns and villages, teaching in their synagogues, proclaiming the gospel of the Kingdom, and curing every disease and illness" (Matthew 9: 35). In the context of the passage, however, it is also noted that when Jesus saw the crowds in need, his heart was moved with "pity" (Matthew 9: 36).

The word *compassion,* in its Latin derivation, is broadly described as meaning "to suffer" with someone, to take on the pain of their burden. The nursing literature on compassion seems to support that understanding in articles dealing with such topics as compassionate caring, empathy/compassion, and compassion for suffering. There are myriad ways to express compassion in nursing such as that described in the first chapter in the parable of compassion for the homeless patient. Without the support of prayer, however, the ability to truly embrace patients' needs, to truly practice compassionate caregiving, will be extremely difficult if not impossible.

A PLACE OF SILENCE IN NURSING

How do we minister compassionately to the wounded Christ in today's complex and stressful health care world? In the previous chapter, I cited the advice of Brother Lawrence of the Resurrection that we, as nurses, try to develop an "oratory of the heart." To do that, to be able to see Jesus in each person for whom we care, we need to find a place of silence in our nursing.

I discovered a wonderful article addressing the concept of silence in an early nursing journal; the author described nurses as "captives of God," and commented: "The nurse, in the midst of her crowded ward, can yet within the innermost mansion of her soul dwell alone with God, in the solitude that lovers seek. In the midst of all the noise of her work she can preserve within herself a place of silence where she can listen to her beloved."[1]

To find this place of silence within is critical to creating a prayerful practice of nursing. Most scholars of prayer discuss the importance of silence as a necessary dimension of a developing prayer life. Wayne Simsic stresses the fact that silence has a calming effect on the mind and heart and allows our prayer life to grow. "Silence," he notes, "is not a thing outside us but an ineffable presence that calls us to prayer."[2] Brother Roger of Taize reminds us that even during those silent times when we feel that we are alone, God is with us. "He is praying within us in the silence of our hearts, in an unvoiced prayer."[3] And Henri Nouwen, while admitting that achieving this inner quiet is not easy, asserts that silence is the core of all prayer: "In the beginning we often hear our own unruly inner noises more loudly than God's voice. This is at times very hard to tolerate. But slowly, very slowly, we discover that the silent time" leads us to prayer.[4]

I agree with Henri Nouwen that achieving a state of inner silence, a prayerful place within, is not easy, especially for those of us whose vocation of caring for the sick seems far more active than contemplative. Sometimes we simply need to accept the "unruly inner noises" and offer these to the Lord as our prayer. A Carthusian novice master described the silence of prayer as a "mystery" and as a gift from God which we cannot force. "Once we have heard this silence, we thirst to find it again [but] we must, however, free ourselves from the idea that we can, of ourselves, reproduce it."[5]

In Chapter 4, I shared the story of a profound personal prayer experience that I had during a weekend visit to a spiritual center. The brief but very intense and prayerful time of being with the Lord was a surprise; it occurred not in the chapel but outdoors, when I was cold and tired and just about ready to pack it in for the night. My spirit soared and my heart was filled with joy at an awareness of God's love and tenderness which I experienced in the silence and solitude of a deserted forest path. I did, of course, as the Carthusian novice master noted, "thirst to find it again," and, because patience does not happen to be one of my best virtues, I thirsted to find it again as soon as possible.

As it happened, the following day the spiritual center I was visiting offered their guests the option of spending an hour of prayer with the community's cloistered Sisters. We were to be introduced to the concept of "centering prayer" (discussed in Chapter 8) and then have silent time to "practice" in the Cloister Chapel. "Wow," I thought considering my earlier prayer experience, "this will be great!" Well, I sort of thought that, at least when I allowed my emotional side, "thirsting" for another deeply prayerful experience, to take over. A small, more reasoned, inner voice did, however, remind me that such silent prayer is a gift from God; not something one can, as noted earlier, "reproduce" at will.

Despite the influence of my rational nature, however, I arrived at the Cloister the next day hoping. One of the sisters gave us a brief explanation of "centering prayer" and then led us to the chapel. The Cloister Chapel, which I had always loved, was small and inviting. It was furnished with great simplicity, much to my personal taste. There were small prayer benches and pillows on the floor; the lights were dimmed and a number of fragrant candles were burning. The ambiance was perfect: silent and prayerful to assist us in entering into a reflective presence before the Lord. I alternately knelt and sat on the floor quietly and prayerfully for about an hour. It was a lovely and peaceful experience but ... you guessed it ... nothing happened. What I mean is, nothing happened emotionally to stir my heart and my spirit as on the previous evening during my solitary forest walk with the Lord; His time and His place are very often not ours.

Was I still praying during that time in the Cloister Chapel? Absolutely. I simply did not, in that prayer experience, have the gift of an emotional or a "feeling" awareness of the presence of the Lord which I had been given earlier. This latter sort of prayer is, however, the more usual kind of encounter with the Lord for most of us. I don't mean dryness or distraction, although that surely does happen at times (as discussed in Chapter 7); but simply the fact that most often our times of prayer are directed by a conscious desire to be with the Lord rather than being the product of or the desire for an emotional high, which may or may not occur.

To get back to the meaning of "silence" for practicing nurses, I have to admit that when I searched the concept in the nursing literature, I found that most articles dealt with the patient's need for times of silence and solitude as a dimension of privacy. No contemporary authors wrote about a nurse's need for personal silence, although two articles did address silence as a dimension of nursing therapy. A *British Journal of Nursing* article reported on the importance of listening, which the author described as "silent communication."[6] And, a U.S. article entitled "Using Therapeutic Silence in Home Healthcare Nursing," concluded that, although it may at times be uncomfortable for the nurse, purposeful silence can be an effective nursing intervention.[7]

The achieving of a "place of silence" in our nursing will need to be a unique and creative process for each of us. It may happen during a drive to work in the morning. I have a friend who told me that she considers her car to be like a small personal chapel, "because," she said "when I'm driving, it's the one time and the one place during my day that I know I can be alone." Places of silence can also be created while waiting in line (which most of us dislike), during periods of gathering for a meeting before the group has assembled, or when moving from place to place in the course of running work-related errands. Whenever, however, and wherever we can create these small places of silence in our hearts, they will provide fertile soil for the inspirations of the Holy Spirit to take root; they are essential to incorporating the concept of spiritual gentleness into the practice of our nursing.

PRAYER AND SPIRITUAL GENTLENESS IN NURSING

"Your adornment should not be an external one ... but rather the hidden character of the heart, expressed in the imperishable beauty of a GENTLE and calm disposition, which is precious in the sight of God."

1 Peter 3: 3

A deeply prayerful minister to the ill and the infirm was the late Cardinal John O'Connor; Cardinal O'Connor, always an advocate for the sick, was particularly loved for his tender ministry to AIDS patients at St. Clare's Hospital in New York. According to numerous anecdotes, the cardinal did not just visit those hospitalized with HIV-related illnesses, he physically cared for them as well, helping with whatever nursing tasks were needed during a visit. And yet, in speaking to a group of health care professionals, the cardinal asserted that what he had learned, following his extensive ministry to those living with HIV infection, was that the most important approach in caring for the sick was to treat patients with spiritual gentleness. This, His Eminence maintained, was more important than "any physical or medical help" a nurse can give.[8]

As I thought and prayed about Cardinal O'Connor's concept of spiritual gentleness, as central to the activity of nursing the sick, I realized that such as approach can only be adopted if one's nursing is centered in and supported by prayer. Thus, I decided to explore the meaning of spiritual gentleness and its relationship to prayer in the theological and nursing literature, and as understood by practicing nurses.

The evangelist Luke has been described as "the scribe of Christ's gentleness"; this title is associated with Luke's emphasis on the mercy and forgiveness of Jesus, for example, Jesus' concern for the poor (Luke 2: 15, the visit of the poor shepherds to Mary and Jesus) and the outcast (Luke 7: 36, the pardon of the woman with the alabaster flask).[9] Throughout the New Testament one finds myriad references to Jesus' gentleness and to the gentleness required of those who follow Him, e.g., "Come to me, all you who labor and are burdened.... Take my yoke upon you and learn from me, for I am meek and humble of heart" (Matthew 11: 28–29); Paul's defense of his ministry which begins: "Now I myself, Paul, urge you through the gentleness and clemency of Christ" (2 Corinthians 10: 1); Paul's exhortation to the Galatian converts on the activity of the Holy Spirit in their lives: "the fruit of the Spirit is love, joy, peace, patience, kindness, generosity, faithfulness, gentleness, self-control" (Letter to the

Galatians 5: 22–23); Paul's first letter to the Thessalonians, in which he noted that the Christian ministers did not seek praise or "impose our weight as apostles of Christ" but rather "were gentle among [the new Christians], as a nursing mother cares for her children" (1 Thessalonians 2: 7); a letter to James that describes true wisdom "from above" as "all pure, then peaceable, gentle, compliant, full of mercy and good fruits" (James 3: 17); and the First Letter of Peter, in which the author addressed the Christian acceptance of suffering: "Always be ready to give an explanation to anyone who asks you for a reason for your hope, but do it with gentleness and reverence" (1 Peter 3: 15–16).

In searching the theological literature, I found two books that focused specifically on the topic of spiritual gentleness: *The Spirituality of Gentleness* by Judith Lechman and *Spirituality and the Gentle Life* by Adrian Van Kaam. Van Kaam related the ability to live a gentle life directly to prayer and the practice of the presence of God: "Awareness of the presence of the Divine instills gentleness in the human soul. That same gentleness seems in turn to deepen awareness of the Presence that evoked this feeling.... The key to a gentle life style ... seems to be a continuous awareness of the Divine Presence."[10] Van Kaam pointed out that the desire and attempt to live gently are supportive of developing a life of prayer: "In living the gentle life style, (one) may discover ... that it becomes easier ... to pray, to meditate, to stay attuned to God's presence. Gentility stills and quiets ... the ego. A silenced ego allows [one] to center ... in Divine ground."[11]

Judith Lechman explained that her search to understand the spirituality of gentleness was derived from Christian Scripture, and she described a paradigm consisting of four stages of gentleness. These stages consist of hearing the call of Christ to gentleness, attempting to learn Christ's ways, moving from belief to action, and entering into a state in which one's life "becomes an expression of gentleness."[12]

Many other spiritual writers address the concept of spiritual gentleness as a characteristic of Christian faith. A great advocate of gentleness, as of prayer, was Francis De Sales who reminded the reader of *Introduction to a Devout Life* to keep in mind the main lesson that Jesus left us: "'Learn of me,' he said, 'that I am gentle and humble of heart.' That says it all," asserted De Sales, "to have a heart gentle toward one's neighbor and humble toward God."[13] Gentleness, from a spiritual perspective, has also been described as: "a fundamental ingredient of Christian character" and a sign of God's creative work in us;[14] "an outward display of true love";[15] "strength under control";[16] "composure in the midst of stress";[17]

and a grace "produced in us by the Holy Spirit."[18] The beatitude "Blessed are the gentle for they will inherit the land" is identified as epitomizing the coincidence of opposites: "One has to be really strong and secure in oneself in order to be gentle. This is not a beatitude for the wishy-washy and faint hearted. There is real power in gentleness."[19]

Recognition of the concept of spiritual gentleness as central to the practice of nursing began in the Nightingale era. An 1854 poem, "The Nightingale's Song to the Sick Soldier," published while Miss Nightingale was in the Crimea, began a stanza with the line "singing light and gentle hands and a nurse who understands."[20] And, Miss Nightingale herself in her 1859 *Notes on Nursing* suggested a gentle approach in noting that "all hustle and bustle is peculiarly painful to the sick."[21] An 1892 nursing textbook observed that, until a few years previously, nursing had been carried out by women of questionable moral character and abilities. The nurse author maintained, however, that incompetent care of the sick must be "incomprehensible" for the trained nurse of the day, "who realizes the responsibility which her position involves, and the daily exercise of gentleness, firmness, and tact, which the successful management of the sick necessitates."[22]

Writing of the spirituality of nursing the sick in 1893, Isabel Hampton stated that "the nurse must have ... self-sacrifice, love of the work, devotion to duty, the courage and coolness of the soldier, the tenderness of the mother";[23] an 1895 nursing text recommended that because the sick are very sensitive to "the state of things around them," a nurse working in the sick room needs to be "quiet, gentle, and patient";[24] and an 1898 text entitled *Practical Points in Nursing* asserted, not only that the nurse should in all cases be "gentle, kind, charitable and patient" but also that the poor person should be "as tenderly nursed as if he were the highest in the land."[25]

In a 1919 book on nursing ethics, it was advised that nurses should acquire a "sensitiveness of touch" which should "at all times be gentle, showing sympathy and tenderness" to the sick;[26] a 1928 text on the same topic also highlighted the importance of gentleness: "Instinctively we feel that a nurse should be gentle ... few defects in a nurse are more quickly noted by patients or observers than the lack of gentleness."[27]

Nurses' writings for the remainder of the twentieth century continued to include the concept of spiritual gentleness as integral to the art and practice of nursing. Some examples include: two 1929 nurse's prayers, one of which ends "How kind and gentle is a nurse's love";[28] the other stating "We bless Thee O God, for [nurses'] gentleness";[29] a 1935 list of "necessary qualifications of a nurse" that includes "sympathy and gentleness";[30] the classic poem of 1954, "To Be a Nurse Is to Walk with God," which ends with an oft-quoted line of the era: "Oh, white capped nurses, so gentle and true, the Great Physician, Christ, is working through you";[31] and, a 1969 geriatric nurse's poem in which the authors asks, in describing the sobs of a frail elder, "can I calm this storm by the touch of a young gentle hand?"[32]

A 1974 *American Journal of Nursing* article on the care of Alzheimer's patients taught that gentleness was considered the most important characteristic of the nurse-patient relationship;[33] and, in 1976, an article devoted to the philosophy of nursing management, in the journal *Supervisor Nurse*, was entitled "Gentleness: An Attribute for Administrators."[34] In the 1980s, gentleness in nurse-patient interactions was highlighted in such articles as "Reaching Julie with a Gentle Touch," a case study of caring for an abused child;[35] and "The Gentle Touch ... Could We, Should We?" which described a project to explore the activities of male nurses functioning in a "gentle caring role."[36]

Finally, a number of nursing publications in the 1990s identified gentleness as an undergirding theme of nursing. "Gentle Persuasion" was recommended in 1992 as the best way to approach an isolated, home-bound patient;[37] a 1993 article spoke of the importance of compassionate and gentle handling of chronically ill patients;[38] a 1997 ethnographic study described nurses' openness as reflected in the use of gentle touch (39); and a 1998 qualitative study of chronically ill children found that the children's coping was notably strengthened by the gentle caring of their nurses.[40]

To determine an understanding of prayerful spiritual gentleness in contemporary nursing, I queried a group of 15 practicing nurses about their perceptions of the term; all had been in nursing for at least five years. I asked the nurses if they would share some thoughts about or experiences with spiritual gentleness in their practice of nursing. The following are some of the descriptions of the meaning of spiritual gentleness articulated by my respondents.

An oncology nurse provided a definition of spiritual gentleness for the Christian nurse:

> Spiritual gentleness is a quality shown by the nurse who believes she has been called to care for others in the way Jesus taught; kindly, nonjudgmentally, and with a soft touch ... the nurse believing she has been "called" is important because it

influences how she cares. It is possible that gentleness can be an automatic, though admirable, action. The qualifier, spiritual, means that the nurse is actively thinking, living spiritually, and even praying, while she is acting.

An adult nurse practitioner related spiritual gentleness to one's relationship to God:

Spiritual gentleness passes from the spiritual center of one human being to another. In order to practice or experience spiritual gentleness, it is imperative for the nurse to be centered on, or one with God. When the nurse is walking with God, opportunities become available to listen, to communicate and provide the spiritual care patients are seeking.... Spiritual gentleness goes hand in hand with hope. This is one of the greatest spiritual gifts we can give to another; spiritual gentleness is alive and passed along when one connects with another and the patient's sense of hope is nourished.

Another adult nurse practitioner highlighted the relationship of spiritual gentleness to caring:

Spiritual gentleness is intertwined with the concept of caring as the core of the nursing model. The word *spiritual* can have meaning that extends along a continuum. For example, it can be considered that caring itself is a spiritual act. On the other end of the continuum is when the nurse directly prays with a patient. Some possible synonyms for spiritual gentleness are spiritual sensitivity, caring, empathy, compassion or healing touch.

A nurse manager and patient educator identified three specific characteristics of spiritual gentleness:

Spiritual gentleness evokes feelings of understanding and acceptance; it is rooted in the frailty of our humanness; spiritual gentleness increases peace and harmony; spiritual gentleness is the basic ingredient of love.

And, finally, a male nurse working with life threatening illness commented:

I personally see spiritual gentleness in nursing as a way to re-connect with my own feelings/beliefs about spirituality and my commitment to the nursing profession. Spiritual gentleness assists me with my own fears about death and dying, and helps me cope with working with patients who have a life threatening, chronic disease.

Several other members of the nursing group queried gave anecdotal reports of spiritual gentleness either experienced or observed in the course of their practice. A male Navy Nurse Corps member shared the following poignant case example:

I worked in an open ward med/surg ICU with a Navy nurse named Mike. Mike was a muscular man with broad shoulders and big strong arms. He had spent several years at sea with the Navy and was the kind of guy you would like to have around if you were in trouble. One afternoon a young mother was transferred to our ICU from another hospital. She had become ill with an atypical pneumonia which had progressed into ARDS (acute respiratory distress syndrome). She arrived intu-bated and with chest tubes and very much afraid. She was to stay with us and remain intubated for a few weeks. While sev-eral nurses cared for her while she was with us, whenever Mike was working he nursed this young mother. And always during Mike's watch the young mother's hair would be washed. It was not that Mike washed her hair; hair washing was a part of normal nursing care, but it was how Mike washed her hair. It was a slow wash with warm water, fre-quently changed, and gentle massage of her scalp with his big hands. And when the washing was done, the drying and combing and arranging of her hair. All of this accompanied by caring conversation by Mike. It seems a simple thing but it left this young mother who was full of tubes and wires, also full of peace. This came to my mind right away as an example of spiritual gentleness.

A geriatric nurse practitioner told a touching story of one of her patient experiences, which she described as exemplifying spiritual gentleness. The patient, her nurse explained, was a 92-year-old female nursing home resident who had stopped eating and begun to lose a significant amount of weight. The patient had severe peripheral vascular disease and was developing multiple decubiti; she never complained, however, and smiled and was cooperative despite her many physical problems. She had no living relatives, and thus, the physician had become her unofficial guardian. Neither the physician, nor the nursing staff wanted to extend their patient's suffering; they wanted her to have a dignified death. The nurse practitioner explained that, after consultation with a social worker and local ombudsman, the team had decided against any extraordinary measures to prolong life; they agreed to deliver only comfort therapeutics and care in the nursing home. The geriatric nurse practitioner reported:

> Within a week she died a peaceful death. The nursing staff had known the woman for 12 years and they were very distressed over the thought that her body would go to the anatomy board, be cremated and end up in an anonymous grave. So, with the spiritual guidance of her physician and nurse caregivers, a memorial service was arranged. A local funeral home donated their services and a cemetery donated a site for her; even a gravestone was provided. I attended the memorial service and as I sat listening to the minister talk about death and our recognizing the significance of death, I was truly touched. I had this overwhelming sense of spiritual gentleness. Only seven people attended the service but that was seven more than might have been there. I think it was spiritual gentleness that brought us to that service.

A pediatric nurse practitioner described the encounter with a mother whose infant had recently died of SIDS, as reflective of spiritual gentleness:

> About three weeks after Christopher's death, his mother, Anna, came to the office with flu symptoms. At the visit, I noticed that Anna was very tearful, and I invited her to come into my office for a minute; she completely broke down. We sat together on the couch, and she told me how difficult it was coping with Christopher's death. Anna pulled a "Mother's Book" photo album from her bag, and we went through the pictures together. The photo's were heartbreaking. Anna said the hardest thing was all the "what might have beens." Our

visit together was only for a short time, but I felt very close to Anna when she left. She gave me a tight hug and told me it was so nice to be able to talk about Christopher with someone who cared. The next week she sent me a note thanking me for our visit. A priest I know once said that spirituality occurs when you get a "glimpse of God." During my short time with Anna, I realized that in moments like this you do get "a glimpse of God," and that is precisely what brings us to nursing; that is spiritual gentleness in nursing.

Finally, a nurse educator described the spiritual gentleness of teaching:

> In 2 Timothy 2–24, Paul speaks of the Gentle Servant "as one who is gentle unto all men, apt to teach and be patient." Working with the undergrad nursing students each semester has really put gentleness into perspective for me. Teaching the students to master the clinical skills, many have had no prior experience, can be a challenge. But upon hearing a student say "thank you for being so gentle and patient in helping me to accomplish this" is so rewarding and, for me, epitomizes the real essence of spiritual gentleness.

In this era of hi-tech, fast-paced health care and health promotion, nurses desperately need to reaffirm their heritage of spiritual gentleness: a heritage rich with the charism of prayerful devotion to caring for the sick; a heritage characterized by tenderness and empathy in ministering to the ill and the infirm. We must never lose sight of the precious treasure that is ours; for each time we care for the "least brother or sister" of His, we care for our Blessed Lord. This is the great gift of our profession of nursing; this is the grace that makes our nursing a prayer; this is the magnificent blessing of spiritual gentleness is nursing.

SILENT SERMONS OF LOVE: THE NURSE'S MINISTRY OF COMPASSION

I truly believe it's appropriate to describe nurses as ministers, "anonymous" ministers admittedly, but spiritual caregivers nonetheless. To carry this vocational dimension of the nurse's role further, I also believe that nurses, as ministers, preach "sermons" of caring. While some nurses may, in fact, verbally share the spirituality of their compassion, many more will, through their caregiving activities, preach "silent" sermons of love. The warmth of a nurse's smile, the kindness of a nurse's care, the tenderness of a nurse's touch, preach daily messages of unending, unconditional, and unequivocal love toward those for whom the nurse is caring.

Marie was 94 years old, and "ready to meet her Maker," she liked to tell her nurses at the long-term care facility where she had resided for the past five years. Most of Marie's friends had already gone home to the Lord, and there really never had been any blood relatives to speak of; Marie "created" family, she said, "wherever" she "lived and worked." She had created a "family" at the nursing home and Katie, a young nurse, was one of her favorite "children."

Not too many young nurses go into gerontological nursing; it does not seem quite as exciting or challenging as the ICU or the emergency room. But Katie was an exception, a very special exception. She had just graduated from a distinguished baccalaureate program in nursing and decided she wanted to work with elders; Katie reasoned: "they could be my own grandmother or grandfather some day!"

Marie and Katie hit it off right from the beginning; they were both Irish, both loved to tease, and neither cared much for "whiners"; they discovered lots of areas of mutual agreement. As Marie grew more fragile, and Katie more acclimated to being a geriatric nurse, their friendship deepened. Some days, after her shift was over, Katie would stay on and just sit at Marie's bedside, so Marie "would feel like she really did have family at the nursing home," Katie explained.

As a damp and dreary fall rapidly turned to winter for the nursing home residents, Marie's health began to fail dramatically. She seemed to be constantly coughing from a chronic bronchitis that the medications just could not seem to get ahold of; then, one day Marie spiked a vicious temp, and her lungs began to fill with fluid. The house physician proposed hospitalization, but Marie would have none of it; this was her home, she said, and she wanted to "die at home."

I loved to watch Marie and Katie holding hands during those final days; the tiny, frail elder, with her snow white hair and parchment-like skin; the beautiful, dark-haired nurse, exuding life and energy from every pore of her strong young body. Katie did so much for her "adopted" grandmother. It wasn't just the "things" she gave her. Oh, of course, Katie often brought in small gifts like a special lotion or cream to soothe Marie's tender skin, or a small container of ice cream to tempt her waning appetite. But what touched my heart most was the tender and gentle way Katie had of nursing her precious patient: her unfailing kindness, and her consistent patience, her continual loving care.

Katie knew that Marie was going to die and admitted that she, Katie, was much more afraid than her friend; she really wanted to be with Marie, but she had never seen a patient die before. Katie wasn't sure if she could do it, that is, until the time actually came. And then, there she was, once anxious Katie, tearfully and tenderly cradling Marie in her arms, while the Chaplain said a final blessing. Katie truly became both a nurse and a minister that day; she preached a magnificent "silent" sermon of love, as she midwifed her beloved patient into eternal life with the Lord.

A NURSE'S PRAYER FOR A COMPASSIONATE HEART

"When [Jesus] … saw the vast crowd, his heart was moved with pity for them, and he cured their sick."
                                                            Matthew 14: 14

"O God, who alone can grace my spirit with the gift of a compassionate heart, teach me to care. Help me to reach out to those who are in pain, to those who are lonely, to those who are afraid. Bless my nursing that I may become an instrument of Your tender understanding and Your love for those I serve. Let me be a vessel of compassion and caring in Your name. Amen.

6 🖼 The Wounded Healer: Prayer and the Problem of Suffering

"Is anyone among you suffering? He should pray."

James 5: 13

THE PRAYER OF A WOUNDED HEALER

The wounds are many, Dear Lord,
    and deep.
I bruise so easily; it's always
    been that way.
Most of the scars have healed,
    or so it seems.
They're barely visible to the
    eye now; but
      to the heart,
   well, that's another
      matter.

Sometimes, when I least suspect,
    an ache begins somewhere
      far down.
It grows into a hurt that
      burns my throat,
   as I try valiantly
    to master the tears
      begging to be
        shed.

I grab for the nearest Band-Aid,
  seeking desperately to stem
    the bleeding; but nothing
      heals except Your love,
        Dear Lord.
      I'm so tired of
        trying to pretend
          it's otherwise.

And, so, I come humbly to You,
  in prayer; a healer wounded
    in heart and in spirit.
      You anoint my scars with
        the Blessed tears of
          Your Son and they
            are transformed
              and
                made beautiful.

Teach me, Dear Lord, to appreciate
  these liberating wounds, which
    open my nurse's heart to the pain
      of my sorrowful and
        suffering patients.

Teach me, Dear Lord, to accept these
  hidden wounds, which help me to
    understand the loneliness of
      my poor and marginalized
        patients.

Teach me, Dear Lord, to cherish these
  tender wounds, which fill me with
    compassion for the anxiety of
      my frightened and
        hopeless patients.

Teach me, Beloved Wounded Healer, to
  learn of You, that I may become
    myself a healer, wounded

> *yet healed, to be for the injured*
>   *an instrument*
>   *of Your healing*
>   *and*
>   *Your love.*

Nurses see suffering, and they see it up close; and they, in turn, suffer with their patients who are in pain. Both Saints Peter and Paul described a blessedness in suffering when given over to the Lord: "Rejoice to the extent that you share in the suffering of Christ, so that when his glory is revealed you may also rejoice exultantly" (1 Peter 4: 13); "I consider that the sufferings of the present time are as nothing compared with the glory to be revealed for us" (Romans 8: 18). Paul also taught that it was the duty of all Christians to "Rejoice in hope, endure in affliction, [and] persevere in prayer" (Romans 12: 12).

PRAYER AND THE PROBLEM OF SUFFERING

As Christians, we are taught that Jesus' passion and death is our example, par excellence, of how suffering can be embraced and transformed. As discussed in Chapter 7, however, it is not easy to follow a crucified Savior; to some, it may not seem very wise either. During my theology studies, I took a course on "Christian Mysticism." Only a small group of us were enrolled in the class so we did a lot of discussing. One day we were reflecting on the previous week's readings about the life of Beatrice of Nazareth. Beatrice was a thirteenth-century Cistercian nun who frequently used to "swoon" in the chapel; she then had to be carried to her room by the other Sisters. Of course we all had a few tongue-in-cheek comments to make about poor Beatrice's swooning. One of my classmates, a psychiatrist, declared that Bea was probably a manic-depressive. I observed that she would never survive in a contemporary religious community, given her chapel fainting performances.

Our poor beleaguered professor tried to inject some reality, and some charity, into our assessment of Beatrice by reminding his recalcitrant students that mystical experiences were considered much more acceptable in the thirteenth century than they are today. We continued to chuckle, nonetheless, over the strangeness of Beatrice and her sufferings. In the midst of our discussion, I happened to glance at a very large crucifix hanging on the wall; exquisitely crafted crucifixes dominated the walls of all of the seminary classrooms. It suddenly struck me that it might seem pretty strange to non-Christians that a group of students would choose to study in a room whose only artistic decoration was the image of a bleeding, thorn-crowned man suffering the agony of death by crucifixion; the image that to us, as Christians, is dearer than life. Suffering is, indeed, embraced in a variety of ways.

But how can we as nurses embrace suffering that is not directly ours but that of our patients? We can pray for them. We can pray with them. And we can be present to prayerfully share in their experiences of suffering in life and in death.

MIRIAM'S TRANSITUS

During the same period of studying theology just described, one of my Franciscan seminarian classmates invited me to a prayer service to celebrate the Feast of Saint Francis of Assisi; he called the service "Transitus." "Huh?" I replied, at my most articulate; "What's a transitus"? "Well," he explained, "actually it's a celebration of Francis' death. We hold the service on the evening before Francis' feast day in order to rejoice in his crossing over, or transitus, from earthly life to eternal life with the Lord." For those of us who believe in eternal life this surely makes sense. It reminded me of my early days in religious life, when we ate the majority of our meals in silence, except for special feast days. Aside from significant religious holidays, however, whenever one of our sisters died, we had a "recreational" or "talk" meal to celebrate her going to God.

Many times in our nursing practice we are not present at the time of a patient's final suffering or "transitus"; we are not able to prayerfully witness their passing to eternal life. One exception, however, is the situation in which a conscious decision to terminate life support is made in a clinical setting. I experienced such a "transitus" about a dozen years ago; I found it to be a blessing and a grace to be with the dying patient and her family; the prayerfulness of the activity led me to the following reflection and prayer:

MIRIAM'S TRANSITUS: A Nurse's Reflection

The goal of the nursing research I
directed was to support critically ill
ventilator patients, and so we included
Miriam in our project.

She was a young forty-something, but the
    degenerative neuro disease had
    devastated her body and her mind.

Miriam's loved ones couldn't let go;
        for a very long time, it seemed.
Then one day it became too much: "We
        can't let her suffer anymore,"
        they said. "It's time."
The physicians and the nurses agreed;
        and the Chaplain.

I received a call from the ICU; "Miriam's
        vent is going to be dc'd at 1 P.M.,"
        I was told, "We thought you'd
        want to be there."
I did, of course, want to be there;
        well sort of.

I'd never witnessed a ventilator being
        discontinued before; I was frightened.
What if Miriam suffers? It could be so
        painful for her and for the family.
        And for me.

The Chaplain led us in a gentle prayer
        of blessing and farewell: "Dear
            Lord, receive Miriam into your loving
            arms that she may be reborn into
                new life, in eternity,
                with You."

So easily the endotrach tube slipped out;
        so softly the ventilator sighed once,
        and was quiet.
We prayed silently and held Miriam in
        our hearts. Her breathing became
            barely a whisper, and, it wasn't
            long, blessedly ceased.

Miriam's earthly mother gathered her
child into her arms and wept; Miriam's
heavenly Father gathered His child
into His arms and rejoiced.
Miriam was home.

A PRAYER FOR DISCONTINUING LIFE SUPPORT

Dear Father in heaven, we are about to give our dear (name) into
your tender and loving care. You know how hard it is for us to let go;
we have loved (her/him) in health and in illness. We have loved
(her/him) in joy and in sorrow; we have loved (her/him) in strength
and in suffering. Our earthly world will never be the same without
(her/him). But now it is time for (name's) heavenly reward; now it is
time for us to surrender (her/him) into Your loving arms. Bring
(name) into the company of the angels and the saints; let (her/him)
live forever in Your tender care and let (her/his) memory continue to
live each day in the hearts of those who loved (her/him). Amen.

PRAYER AND EMOTIONS IN NURSING: THE LAMP IS HEAVY

Most spiritual writers consider the concept of one's emotions or feelings as a relevant dimension of prayer. Emotions occurring in or around
prayer may be positive, as the example of "feeling" God's presence and
love which I described in Chapter 5; they may be negative relating to
anger at or frustration with God for some perceived offense or unmet
need. One can also have feelings of anxiety, fear, or guilt related to our
relationship or lack of relationship with the Lord. Jesuit William Barry
asserts that if we want to develop a relationship with God we must be
willing to share our emotions and feelings as well as our thoughts.[1] It has
been reported that "the early Christians were not at all afraid of being
emotional in prayer";[2] and that "when we hold nothing back from God,
we eventually come to see that He has been holding nothing back from
us."[3] Related also to including emotions in prayer are using both intu-
ition, or the right-brain "being" side of our nature;[4] and imagination,
which can "open us up to the mystery of God's transforming presence
within us."[5]

The easy part, for me at least, of incorporating emotion into prayer
is the use of positive emotions; I delight in "feeling" the joy and the peace

and the comfort of the gifts of God and of the presence of God in my life and in the lives of others. It's easy to pray happily and gratefully about those things. It's much harder to talk to the Lord about my pain or my anger or my frustration. It just doesn't seem appropriate to bring up negative thoughts or feelings in prayer. Somehow I think that if I don't talk to God about things that are painful to discuss, maybe He won't know what I'm feeling. That is surely a very foolish perception if I really believe, as I say, that God is the center of my life and knows me even better than I know myself.

A nurse friend, who is much wiser than I, shared a good example of using negative emotion in prayer. She was describing the pain of a patient of hers who had been diagnosed with advanced ovarian cancer; she was a young mother with school-age children. The patient confessed that she was very angry with God about her illness and could no longer pray at all. My friend told her gently that she understood why she might feel angry at God, but she advised her, "don't hold it in; you don't have to carry this burden alone. Tell God how angry you are; yell at Him if you want to. God has very strong shoulders. He can take it." My friend's patient told her later that the angry emotional prayer had provided a breakthrough; she could now pray and cry and be angry, yet she had also regained her faith that God was listening to her and loving her, and that He would be with her in whatever she had yet to endure.

When I hear nursing stories like this one, I realize how really heavy a nurse's lamp is some days. As suggested earlier, we can pray for and with our patients; we can listen to them and advise them; we can be present in their times of need. It's almost impossible, however, not to take on some of their pain, which must then be included in our own prayer life, in our own relationship with the Lord. And this is what we often neglect to do in prayer. Think about some recent experience in your hospital, your clinic, your school of nursing, or a patient's home, when you felt deeply a patient, family, or student's personal suffering. Probably you talked about the situation with a close friend or family member—someone who would understand, and care, and share with you a little the burden of suffering you yourself were experiencing. But did you speak about your pain, in prayer, with the Lord?

Personally, I'm sometimes guilty of thinking, if I'm dealing with a very difficult problem, that I'm just too distracted to pray, that I'm so concerned about whatever situation has captured my attention that I just can't be "recollected" or "prayerful" right now. I tend to think: "I'll pray later, when I'm feeling up to it." Not a good strategy. Later may never come, or if it does, I have carried a heavy emotional burden alone for a long time before I finally get around to laying it at the feet of my Lord and my God and asking for help. He waits for us to bring Him our pain, our distraction, and our dryness just as anxiously as He waits for our love and our adoration. That is the consummate blessing of a prayerful relationship with the Lord.

DISTRACTION AND DRYNESS IN PRAYER

I have spent a lot of time exploring books on prayer during the past few years; and virtually all of the spiritual writers in the area include a chapter, or at least a portion of a chapter, on the problems of "distraction" and/or "dryness." Pierre Wolff suggests that we have two kinds of distraction: silly and serious.[6] By silly distractions, he means imaginative thoughts or concerns about day-to-day issues that pop into our heads while we are attempting to pray or meditate. Many years ago, I confessed to a novice mistress that I had spent most of a morning meditation period in chapel worrying about how to insert a 36-inch zipper into a partially made garment bag; I had been assigned to create the bag as a Christmas gift for one of our superiors. I think my novice mistress had quite a difficult time keeping a straight face as she gently advised me to try and restrict my seamstress activities to the sewing room instead of bringing them to chapel. Serious distractions are those that are objectively much more important in our lives such as the terminal illness of a parent or the recent death of a close friend. Peter Kreeft, in his book *Prayer for Beginners* promises that anyone who tries seriously to pray will have distractions: even the saints, he notes "had wandering minds."[7]

Dryness, or a lack of emotion or feeling in prayer, is often related to the concept of the "dark night of the soul" described by the great Saint John of the Cross. In this context, dryness is seen as "intrinsic" to each person's spiritual journey;[8] and a "good and healthy sign of real interior growth."[9] The suffering associated with dryness in prayer is also related to the Gospel message of Jesus: "If anyone wants to follow me, let him ... take up his Cross (Matthew 16: 24); and "Unless a grain of wheat falls to the earth and dies, it remains only a grain" (John 12: 24).[10]

Describing the benefits of distraction in prayer, Mary Clare Vincent, OSB asserts that "distractions are not only inevitable, they are indispensable."[11] Vincent's point is that distractions help us to recognize our own weakness and dependence upon God; they also provide the opportunity to refine our faithfulness to prayer even as we struggle.[12] Periodic dryness can be very fruitful because during such times "our prayer is likely to be most unselfish, most God-centered" as we continue to persevere in prayer through such feelings as apathy or emptiness.[13]

Despite the difficulties associated with distraction and dryness, perhaps one of the most painful experiences for a person of faith is the condition of unanswered prayer. Richard Foster calls unanswered prayer "one of the most troubling issues of petitionary prayer."[14] Foster suggests, however, that there may be several reasons for our perceived lack of response which we need to consider from God's point of view: Sometimes the answer we wish for would not be in the best interest of our spiritual growth; possibly the answer to our prayer could be detrimental to others; or we may be asking for a deeper reality that God sees and we do not, resulting in the fact that a prayer of petition may indeed have been answered but we simply do not recognize the answer.[15] Pierre Wolff notes that we must remember the passage from Isaiah in which the Lord stated: "My thoughts are not your thoughts" (55: 8). If, Wolff adds, we really believe that God hears our prayers when we call out to him, we must also believe that "one way or another" our requests truly are granted.[16]

For us, as nurses, I think that the topics of distraction, dryness, and unanswered prayer are particularly difficult, because we are used to achieving our goals; nurses are primarily "do-ers" rather than "be-ers." We have been educated from early nursing courses that assigned tasks must be accomplished and accomplished well; our patients' lives may depend on it. Thus, it is not easy to simply wait; to simply, as asked by the Lord: "Be still and know that I am God." That, however, is precisely what we must do when we experience the kinds of prayer hindrances described above. We must put aside our goal-oriented mentality, surrender our needs and desires to God, and accept that so often His time and His will are not ours. This is the key to faithfulness in developing a prayer life and in developing a relationship with God. This is the faith that will carry us through on the darkest days when we feel lonely and wounded, that will allow us to become ourselves wounded healers.

PRAYER OF A NURSE WHO IS WOUNDED: A NURSE'S SERMON ON THE MOUNT

I have written before about the nurse as a wounded healer;[17] as a gifted healer, whose wounds may be used for the good of those she cares for. I truly believe, for a nurse especially, that woundedness is a gift, for "to be wounded is to be human; to be wounded is to be vulnerable; to be wounded is to be a reflection of the consummate wounded healer, Jesus of Nazareth, the touchstone of our hope and the center of our lives."[18] Our patients come into our care at their most human, their most vulnerable, and their most wounded. A nurse who understands is a patient's greatest blessing; compassionate understanding is the greatest gift we can bring to the practice of our nursing.

To bring our personal woundedness into our nursing, however, is a delicate mission and can only be accomplished by prayer and in prayer. Woundedness of any sort is difficult to acknowledge; it is difficult for caregivers especially. We need to feel strong; we need to feel capable; we need to feel on top of things. These are all good emotions and surely positive characteristics for a nurse. But often it is precisely from our places of vulnerability, our places of woundedness, that our deepest compassion and caring for others are derived. It is for the ability to use these gifts of woundedness in our ministry that we must pray.

A Nurse's Sermon on the Mount

Florence Nightingale once wrote that "A good nurse should be the 'Sermon on the Mount' in herself."[19] That's a pretty powerful call to ministry, even coming from a nursing pioneer deeply imbued with the spirit of Christian commitment and caring. If we truly take Florence's maxim to heart, it means we, as nurses, should bless the poor in spirit, comfort those who mourn, support the weak, provide justice for those who are marginalized, be merciful to those in need of mercy, encourage purity of heart, promote peace, and protect the persecuted. Only acknowledgment of our own woundedness in prayer, I think, can help us to understand and accept such a ministry to those with so many and such varied wounds.

The challenges facing the nursing profession today can, at times, seem overwhelming. One of the things that helps my prayer life when I get stressed over too many tasks, too little time, and too few resources, is to meditate on the struggles and the accomplishments of great saints who have cared for the sick before me; the men and women on whose shoulders we contemporary nurses now stand. Although she would probably be most unwilling to accept the label "saint," one of my twentieth-century heroines is the French military nurse Genevieve de Galard-Terraube, who was labeled by the world "the Angel of Dien Bien Phu."

Genevieve was assigned to serve in a Vietnam military field hospital during the French occupation of Hanoi in the early 1950s; one of her duties as an air flight nurse was to accompany wounded soldiers on evacuation flights from an underground fortress near the front lines at Dien Bien Phu. On one such trip, Genevieve's plane was shot down and the pilot and passengers were grounded; Genevieve was now the only woman at the front. Although her superior officers attempted to protect her, Genevieve refused to stay in the safety of the fortress; she frequently risked her life, amidst mortar shelling, to care for wounded soldiers on the battlefield. She also refused numerous opportunities to be liberated, choosing instead to stay with her patients.

After the war, Genevieve received many medals, including the French Croix De Guerre and the Legion of Honor, as well as numerous other awards and accolades; she was esteemed throughout the world as a model of courage and commitment. A New York City ticker-tape parade was held to honor her on a visit to the United States in 1954; at the time, she was presented with the Medal of Freedom by President Dwight D. Eisenhower. When interviewed, Genevieve described an atmosphere of deep religious feeling among the soldiers for whom she cared, and she stated that she herself always trusted that God had been there to protect her. Clearly she was a woman of prayer; it was reported that "her most valued possession" was a rosary given to her by the Holy Father as a token of his "high regard for her courageous charity."[20] In the end, however, Genevieve de Galard-Terraube, the "Angel of Dien Bien Phu," insisted that she had only done "what any nurse would do!"

A NURSE'S PRAYER FOR COURAGE IN SUFFERING

"I have told you this so that you might have peace in me. In the world you will have trouble, but take COURAGE, I have conquered the world."

John 16: 33

Lord Jesus, wounded healer of our hearts, teach me to embrace suffering. This is not an easy prayer; I get very afraid. Sometimes it seems "my soul is sorrowful unto death" (Matthew 26: 38). Only You whose "sweat became as drops of blood falling on the ground" can be my teacher and my guide. I don't understand sickness and sorrow. I hurt with those in pain; I want to take away their suffering. I long to cry out with You "Father, if You are willing, take this cup away." Bless me, Lord Jesus, with the courage and the love to complete Your prayer: "still not my will but Yours be done" (Luke 22: 39–42). Amen.

7   The Journey to Jerusalem: Prayer and a Healing Ministry

"Therefore ... pray for one another, that you may be healed."
James 5: 16

VERONICA: A Nurse's Meditation

Standing at the fringes of the crowd,
   she feels the restlessness.
She shades her eyes from the hot Jerusalem sun
   and peers down the road;
It's so dry and dusty, she can't see anything
   but she senses His coming.
Her heart begins to beat fast and her
   temples pound.
How could they do this to her dear and
   gentle Rabbi; the One who taught
     her to love in His Father's
      name?

Then, over the rise of a hill, she catches
   the first painful glimpse.
The soldiers surround Him; as if He had
   the desire, or even the strength
     to run!
The Cross is fearful; its wood so heavy,
   its beams so rough.
He can barely drag it down the path; only
   the young, strong arms of Simon make

97

the humiliating procession
possible.

As He draws near she sees the beautiful
face; now caked with the dirt of the
streets and blood from the cruel
beating.
Crimson droplets trickle into His loving
eyes; her King is crowned with brambles
and thorns, not with gold and jewels.
Her heart breaks and her soul weeps bitter
tears; she feels so helpless.

She has no towel or cloth to wipe the precious
wounded face; only a poor woman's veil,
simple muslin, but soft and clean; put
on that very afternoon to preserve
humility before the eyes of her Lord.
Modesty is no longer relevant; now she must
bare her head to blot the blood and tears
from those same beloved eyes.
She is rewarded with the Blessed image of
the Divine Son of God.

I see him stumble into the ER, leaning
heavily on his comrade's arm.
"He's homeless," his friend from the
family of the streets reports:
"They beat him up, those young punks,
just because he's old."

His body is caked with the dirt of the
streets, and blood from the cruel
beating.
His eyes are moist with unshead tears; alive
with the pain of loneliness and fear.
I wash the gentle, weathered face with a
clean, soft towel, and I think of
Veronica.
I am rewarded with the Blessed image of
the human Son of God.

Benedictine Scripture scholar Jerome Kodell asserts that Jesus' Journey to Jerusalem reflected the "fulfillment of God's plan" for his life and provided direction and inspiration for all Christian followers to come: "We find ourselves on the way toward Jerusalem with the Lord. But the march to glory, as Jesus has already warned, is a path through suffering. The disciples must expect to be treated no better than the Master."[1] We, as nurses, encounter this Journey to Jerusalem in many dimensions, not only in our own lives, but also in those of our patients and families. And, as we travel the path that Jesus trod, we have precious opportunities to share in his healing ministry to those in need. Nurses may model the hands-on care of the holy woman Veronica or the young Simon of Cyrene; we may become engaged in some or all of the way stations that Our Lord encountered on his journey to the Cross; we may be involved in a healing ministry of presence through our empathy and compassion for those who are suffering. Ultimately, however, nurses' Journeys to Jerusalem, our healing ministries, must be grounded in prayer: prayer of trust in the great and tender love of the Father; prayer of desire to live deeply the Gospel message of his Divine Son; and prayer of hope for the inspiration of the Blessed Spirit of God who will guide our hands and purify our hearts.

PRAYER AND THE NURSE'S JOURNEY TO JERUSALEM

Several years ago I participated in a challenging course on the theology of the Christian church. The class consisted of a fairly large group of clergy and lay people who planned to work in the area of pastoral ministry. One particular evening our class members were extremely gregarious; there was an unusual amount of talking and laughter as we waited for class to begin. I am not sure if it was our high spirits, or simply the inspiration of the Holy Spirit, but something moved our professor to begin her lecture with a Christian principle that remains etched in my heart to this day. After a brief opening prayer, she looked around at the assembled students and observed: "You have all come here with enthusiasm and excitement at the prospect of serving the Lord, at the thought of working in ministry; that's wonderful, but I need to remind you that, if you plan to follow Jesus, there's a small matter of a 'Journey to Jerusalem' that goes along with that walk!"

Our class responded with what seemed like a collective intake of breath. We were reminded both individually and as a group that we follow a crucified Lord. We follow a Savior who embraced suffering and shame because of his love for the world. We follow Jesus of Nazareth, whose ministry was to give up His earthly life that others might have the gift of eternal life. And, as our professor gently yet graphically reminded us, he expects no less of his followers. Our leader and Lord is the same Jesus who taught: "If anyone wishes to come after me, he must deny himself and take up his cross daily and follow me" (Luke 9: 23); "Whoever loves his life, / loses it, and whoever hates his life in this world, will preserve it for eternal life. Whoever serves me must follow me" (John 12: 25–26); and "Go, sell what you have, and give to the poor ... then come, follow me" (Mark 10: 21).

I have always been drawn to Jesus in the passion and death he embraced in his humanity; perhaps that's because, as a nurse, I have witnessed so much suffering humanity in the experiences of my patients. But, even more than that, I think it's because, being possessed of a romantic Irish temperament, I am somewhat "in love" with love. And, I can't imagine any more deeply loving life than that of Jesus, the Christ, my Lord and my Savior. I want mightily to follow the path set out by this greatest lover of all time. It is not, I have learned, an easy road.

Personally, I seem to do fairly well at the beginning of the "journey"; I like sharing the Gospel message of Jesus, or at least I like to try; I have lots of energy, and the excitement of the trip buoys me up. It's as the walk with Jesus progresses that my problems begin. As I move deeper into the real meaning of the journey; when I glimpse, even in the far distance, the lights of Jerusalem, I start to experience a tightness in my throat. When I begin to envision the humiliation, the pain, and God forbid, the hill of Calvary, which I may have to encounter, my heart constricts; I want to start backpedaling, away from Jerusalem, away from the Cross, as fast as I can. This journey is not for the faint of heart. It is a journey that takes a courage and a love and a strength that can be found only in prayer and in listening with one's heart to the Word of God. For it is only through hearing God's holy word in the Scriptures that we are inspired not only to take up but also to continue our Journey to Jerusalem; and it is only through receiving God's strength and God's love, from kneeling at his feet in prayer, that we are able to tread the path which the Master trod.

When we look at Jesus' teaching in the Scriptures, even in the powerful passages cited earlier, we see, however, that his teachings contain not only great challenges but also great rewards for those who would dare embark on this faith-filled journey: "For whoever ... loses his life for my sake, will save it" (Luke 9: 24); "The Father will honor whoever serves me" (John 12: 26); and "You will have treasure in heaven" (Mark 10: 21).

When we read these Scriptures meditatively, our hearts cannot help but be moved by the magnificent gifts that Jesus promised as reward for the risk of following him. We will "save" our lives; the father will "honor" us; and we shall have "treasure in heaven." For myself, however, it is only when I take such thoughts and go humbly before the Lord in prayer that my soul is touched, that my strength, my courage, and my love are renewed. As discussed earlier, prayer is a gift and a grace. We cannot force it; we cannot control it. We can, nonetheless, place our bodies and our spirits in a posture to seek and to receive God's precious gift of love. Thus, we must indeed ask without ceasing: Lord, teach us to pray.

Benedict Groeschel has observed that there is no right or wrong way of "listening at prayer."[2] In the final chapter some "methods" of placing oneself in a posture of prayer are discussed, but it is important to remember that, for a nurse, prayer may take on many and varied faces. Prayer in action became a vibrant and living reality when reflected in the conduct of Jesus' disciple Veronica, who is often considered a prefigure of the nurse.

VERONICA: PREFIGURE OF THE NURSE

While exploring the early nursing literature to learn whether the concept of prayer was identified with the role of the professional nurse, I began to notice a number of writings in which the Christian woman Veronica was described as a prefigure of the nurse. Veronica, or Saint Veronica as she is described by many, is a historical figure whom legend identifies as having wiped the wounded face of Jesus during his agonizing journey to Calvary. That compassionate act of Veronica was often associated in the literature with discussions of the prayer life of a nurse.

In a 1939 editorial in *The Trained Nurse and Hospital Review,* it was reported that at a talk given at The Catholic University of America's new school of nursing by the university rector, Veronica was cited as exemplar for practicing nurses. "Veronica, who in seeking to comfort the suffering Christ, wiped his face and found on the towel not blood but the imprint of the love of God."[3] A 1953 meditation entitled "The Nurse's Mass" included the nurse author's spiritual yearning: "Even as Veronica wiped the perspiring face of Our Lord, so may I soothe the fevered brow and wash away the tears, and may my reward be His image in my heart."[4] In two 1954 papers in *The Catholic Nurse,* Veronica is envisioned as the nurse's role model. One article, "Modern Veronicas," reported that the priest author has witnessed nursing "Veronicas figuratively wipe the bleeding face of the mystical body of Christ in dying cancer patients."[5] In the second paper, the author suggested that prayer is central to every nursing act and posed the question: "Would you not say that Veronica, who walked along the sorrowful road to Calvary" and wiped the face of Christ, "would you not call that a prayer?"[6] And describing the nurse again as a "modern Veronica," Albert Mayer advised in a 1958 article that all nurses show their patients the "sympathy, tender thoughtfulness and compassion which Veronica showed to Christ on the Via Dolorosa."[7] He notes: "To be a modern Veronica ... means that we are willing to translate our pity and compassion into concrete assistance and practical help as Veronica did. The Passion of Christ is being hourly renewed in the sufferings of those about us. To be a modern Veronica means not to be blind to these sufferings."[8]

Commentaries published in the early 1960s reflect a similar theme. For example, it was observed that on Jesus' walk to Calvary "no one ... offered him physical comfort except Veronica"; and questions were raised: "Could it be that she was experienced in giving care to those who suffered? Could we [nurses] not continue, by acts of love, to mystically 'wipe the holy face'?";[9] and, "Veronica braved the insults of the mob and the soldiers to wipe [Jesus'] blood stained Holy Face. She is the model of our public health nurses."[10] Finally, in her 1973 history of the profession, Josephine Dolan pointed out that nursing practice was fostered, from its inception, by Christian values and by the witness of individuals such as Veronica who "wiped the agonized face of Christ" and who "will be recorded for all time for their example in comforting the afflicted."[11]

THE LEGEND

But who, really, was this woman we call "Veronica"; this legendary woman who is believed to have risked her life in one grand act of compassion and courage, an action that would be remembered and honored for 2000 years? She stood "at the fringes of the crowd" her heart broken and bleeding. She had no thought for her own safety. She had no fear of the Roman soldiers' revenge. Only He mattered, her beloved Rabbi. Would any one of us have been so brave? And so exquisitely loving?

The legend of Veronica wiping the face of Jesus has no accepted scriptural reference. An apocryphal (from the Greek *apocrypha* meaning hidden) text, an early writing never accepted into the canon of Christian Scripture, "The Gospel of Nicodemus," discusses a woman with a 12-year hemorrhage who was cured by touching the hem of Jesus' robe (Matthew

9: 20–22); the woman is assigned the name *Veronica*, "And a woman called Bernice [Latin: Veronica] crying out from a distance said: 'I had an issue of blood and I touched the hem of his garment, and the issue of blood, which had lasted twelve years, ceased'" (Luke 8: 43–48).[12]

In a nineteenth-century commentary on the apocryphal gospels, a chapter entitled "The Story of Veronica" seems to support the brief passage in the Gospel of Nicodemus by suggesting that Veronica, "having been healed by Jesus," wished to "erect a monument to him" and sought permission from King Herod to do this.[13] And in a French text on Christian apocrypha, *La Vengeance de Nostre-Seigneur*, a passage cited from a fourteenth-century French Bible, loosely translated, relates a narrative of Our Lord passing before a holy woman named Veronica. And when the woman saw the Lord in his great suffering, the passage continues, she began to weep and offered Jesus her veil to wipe his bleeding face. Then the image of Jesus appeared on the veil.[14]

Although a number of variations appear among the stories of Veronica in the literature, the central elements of the legend, which first emerged in the fourteenth century,[15] are similar. Veronica is clearly remembered as a woman who was present in the crowd following Jesus as he carried his Cross to Calvary. Seeing her Rabbi painfully perspiring, bleeding, and bent from the weight of the Cross, the woman identified as Veronica is believed to have stepped forward and wiped his face with her veil. As a reward for her courage and compassion, Veronica's veil is said to have been imprinted with the blessed image of Jesus' suffering face. In advocating a lesson to be learned from the imprinting of Jesus' face on Veronica's veil, it is asserted: "As always nothing is offered to Him that is not returned a hundredfold."[16]

Minor details of the legend vary such as whether Veronica wiped Jesus' face with a towel or a head covering; the most frequently used terms for the cloth employed, however, are veil, scarf, or kerchief. After the report of this one great act of love, there is little information about Veronica. Some versions of the legend suggest that she brought the veil to Rome and used it to cure the Emperor Tiberius of a serious illness.[17] Veronica is variously identified as having been the wife of Zaccheus; the wife of a Roman Officer; or Martha, one of the sisters of Lazarus. Virtually all commentaries on the legend confirm that the woman believed to have comforted Jesus in his anguish was assigned the name *Veronica* because of the miraculous imprint of Jesus' face on the cloth; *Veronica* is derived from the Latin words *vera* and *icon* meaning true image.[18] To this day an ancient cloth, believed by many to bear the imprint of the Lord's face, is preserved in St. Peter's Church in Rome where it may be venerated by the faithful.[19]

The historical figure Veronica is most often honored by Christians who employ the practice of meditating on the "The Way of the Cross" as a dimension of their prayer life. The concept of prayerfully meditating on the 14* key occurrences during Jesus' Passion came into common practice around the time of the Middle Ages. The "Way of the Cross" begins with the first incident of Jesus' Passion narrative, his condemnation to death, and concludes with the entombment of the Lord's body. Other occurrences highlighted in the meditations are several falls under the weight of the Cross; Jesus' meeting of his mother and other women followers; Simon's assistance in carrying the Cross; and, the Crucifixion, death, and removal of Jesus' body from the Cross.

The sixth occurrence or "station" of "The Way of the Cross" describes the compassion of Veronica in wiping the face of Jesus. Many commentaries speak to the meaning of the sixth station of the Cross for contemporary Christians. One observes: "Veronica abandoned the safety of the crowd and took Jesus something of her clothes ... she gave of her clothing; she gave of herself."[20] Another suggests that Veronica, in her caring and compassion, is the real model of the Christian, that she stands as "a true image of what Christ asked all men and women to become in his name."[21] And a third points out that we do not have to have lived in the time of Jesus to "replicate" Veronica's courage and devotion: "Each person we meet provides an opportunity to put into practice Christ's words: 'In as much as you did this to one of the least of my brothers and sisters, you did it to me.'"[22]

Finally, in a beautifully poignant commentary on "The Way of the Cross," spiritual writer Caryll Houselander observed that it was compassion that drove Veronica to step out bravely and act, and it is compassion that inspires the "Veronicas of today" to overcome their anxieties and fears and reach out to those in need. First among these "Veronicas," the author cited "Nurses who comfort the dying in hospitals ... who go into the homes of the sick and the poor to serve."[23] Ultimately, Houselander asserted, it is not only the healing of the physical wounds to which these "Veronica's" attend, but it is also to the care of emotional and spiritual needs that tender compassion leads them.[24] This is the gift of Veronica of history; this is the gift of the nurse as a "modern Veronica."

---

*In recent years, the Resurrection of Jesus from the dead has been identified by some as a 15th station of the Cross, to complete the Lord's Passion experience.

THE NURSE: A MODERN VERONICA

Having explored the legend of Veronica from the perspective of both Christian and nursing literature, I began to wonder if the twenty-first-century nurse could accept the Veronica of history as a prefigure or role model. Could contemporary nurses identify with the label "modern Veronica"? What does it really mean for us, as nurses, to wipe the face of a suffering patient? Have we present day nurses the courage and the "tender compassion" that Caryll Houselander perceived in our earlier counterparts? I sought the answers to these questions from the most reliable source I could think of—the experiences of young practicing nurses.

Before exploring the nurses' experiences, however, I briefly examined the literature on the nursing procedure of "washing a patient's face"; I wanted to find out if nurse educators, both past and present, perceived a spiritual or compassionate theme associated with the activity.

Washing a Patient's Face: The Nursing Literature

In her classic 1859 work, *Notes on Nursing*, Florence Nightingale taught that a significant amount of relief and comfort was observed at the "sick bed" after a patient's face had been washed.[25] Nightingale explains that this comfort is not simply from the cleansing but indicates that a patient's "power" has been strengthened because "something oppressing was removed."[26] Isabel Hampton Robb, writing in 1906, maintained that washing a patient's face could greatly relax and even energize the person to cope with a stressful situation.[27] And Amy Pope and Virna Young asserted in 1934 that washing a patient's face helped to relieve the fatigue and strain experienced by those "who have been subjected to worry, excitement or other causes of excessive nervous stimulation."[28] Nurse authors writing in the middle and later twentieth century suggest additional benefits of washing a patient's face such as: refreshment of mind and body;[29] sedation;[30] and overall relaxation.[31] A contemporary nursing fundamentals text explains that because of the importance of the skin as the body's first line of defense, the cleansing of a patient's face of foreign materials is a significant activity in the practice of nursing.[32]

From the literature just cited, the "spiritual" importance of wiping or washing a patient's face can only be inferred. However, comments related to such issues as comfort, strengthening of power, removal of something oppressing, energizing to cope with stressful situations, refreshment of mind and body, and care of the body's first line of defense broadly support the acceptance of a "spiritual" dimension within this physical ministry of caring. Veronica, as earlier described, did indeed seem to have the mind and heart of a nurse; she reached out in the only way she could think of to attempt to ease the suffering of her beloved Rabbi and Lord, Jesus of Nazareth. From the perceptions of the nurse educators cited, it would seem that Veronica's act of care may have greatly comforted the Lord not only physically but also spiritually.

Washing a Patient's Face: The Practicing Nurses

I asked a group of 15 newly practicing nurses to respond to two specific questions derived from the concept of Veronica as a model for the nurse: first, whether they perceived any kind of spiritual component to the nursing activity of washing/wiping a patient's face; and second, whether their own nursing experiences of wiping/washing a patient's face had ever provided the opportunity for developing a spiritual relationship or bond with the patient.

All 15 nurses interviewed agreed (8 "strongly agreed" and 7 "agreed") that there was a spiritual dimension to washing/wiping a patient's face. In regard to personal experiences of washing/wiping patients' faces leading to a spiritual bonding between patient and nurse, 11 nurses agreed (2 "strongly agreed" and 9 "agreed"), 3 were uncertain, and only 1 nurse disagreed. Thus, contemporary practicing nurses do, in theory and in practice, support the concept of Veronica as prefigure and role model.

I also asked the nurses to respond in narrative form to a third, open-ended question to flesh out responses on the earlier items. The question was, "Please describe the spiritual meaning, for you, of the nursing activity of washing/wiping a patient's face (you may wish to use a case example of a face-washing experience with a particular patient)." The responses, from which the following examples are drawn, made me feel blessed to be a nurse:

> Washing a patient's face makes me think of Jesus telling his disciples "Whatever you do for the least of my people, you do for me." This is just one way, through one small gesture, that I may do as I would for Jesus"; "When I wash someone's face all of the normal boundaries are dissolved. Their need and my care create a spiritual relationship. To do this out of love and respect is a very beautiful connection between two human beings: "For whoever does this for the least of these, does so for Me";

Washing a patient's face is very special. When a person allows you to serve them in this manner it can be very humbling for both the nurse and the patient. Just as Christ washed the feet of others, I feel the same sentiment of washing my patients' faces;

Something spiritual comes over me when I wash a patient's face; there is a deep feeling of trust from that patient;

Before washing a patient's face there is a kind of "stranger" relationship between the patient and the nurse but after the act a spiritual bond does take place;

To wash a person's face may seem like a little thing but it is the little things done with great love that make a difference with God;

I had the experience of washing a dying patient's face in the ICU. I felt it was the most caring thing I could have done for him because he passed away in about an hour; it was a spiritual action for me;

The action of washing a patient's face is spiritual because it means that you are caring for the inner person also. It makes the person feel respected and loved by God; it's a gift for the nurse and patient;

Washing a face shows the patient how much you care about their comfort and brings you closer to the true personality. That's when the spiritual part comes in; the reverence for their life;

Washing a patient's face helps them to see and feel better; just like the manner in which people should treat each other. It can be like washing the face of God.

In looking at the nurses' reflections on the spirituality of washing a patient's face, two characteristics emerge that were also central to the caring ministry of Saint Veronica: courage and anonymity.

Courage

In his first letter to the Corinthians, Paul exhorted the young community: "Be on your guard, stand firm in the faith, be courageous, be strong. Your every act should be done with love" (1 Corinthians 16: 13). Veronica beautifully modeled the courage of love in stepping forth out of a crowd, and braving the possible ire of the Roman guards, to minister to Jesus. The tender wiping or washing of a patient's face may take courage on a nurse's part, also, as reflected in such comments as "washing a patient's face ... can be humbling"; "Before washing a patient's face there is a kind of 'stranger' relationship"; "washing a dying patient's face ... was the most caring thing I could have done"; and "when I wash a patient's face all the normal boundaries are dissolved." Crossing usual interactional boundaries, approaching a stranger, caring for a dying patient, and being humbled are courageous activities; they are prayerful, spiritual activities that practicing nurses carry out each day. The spirituality of such courage is poignantly described by Joyce Rupp who observed "Courage does not mean just gritting our teeth for an endurance test.... Courage means ... believing that we can make it, not on our own power ... but on the Divine Power that is always available if we ask for it."[33] This is the gift of prayer, always available for the support of our nursing practice.

Anonymity

In the end, I believe that one of the most distinctive connections between the legendary Veronica and a practicing nurse is the characteristic of anonymity. As noted earlier, we believe that Veronica may have been "the woman with the hemorrhage" of scripture (Luke 8: 43–48), but we do not know for certain. She has also been identified as, possibly, having been several other historical figures of the New Testament. All that has come to us, in legend, is the fact that a magnificently caring and courageous woman followed her heart and stepped away from the security of the crowd to perform an act of love that would be remembered and honored for centuries to come.

The ministrations of love which nurses carry out are also often anonymous. In a chronicle of contemporary nursing entitled *Life Support: Three Nurses on the Front Lines*,[34] journalist Suzanne Gorden explored the concept of anonymity in nursing. Gorden cites as examples the recovering cardiac surgery patient or the cancer survivor who may "extol" the greatness of (his/her) surgeon or oncologist but, she adds: "what nurses did for these individuals will rarely be mentioned."[35] Yet, the author notes, it was the nurse who calmed the cardiac patient's pre-op anxiety, and it was the nurse who held the head of the oncology patient "wracked with nausea."[36] Gorden explains this anonymity by describing nurses as secret sharers: "Even though (nurses) are patients' lifelines during illness, when control is restored, the residue of [the patient's] anxiety and mortality clings to them like dust and [they] flee the memory."[37]

The latter comment by Gorden sparked an immediate connection with a personal experience in my own clinical practice. Some years ago, I spent many hours at the bedside of a patient undergoing a series of vicious and prolonged chemotherapy treatments for a cancer diagnosis. After the course of chemo was over, and the patient became well, she seemed to significantly distance herself from me. Each time we had an opportunity to interact, I felt a sense of reserve on my former patient's part. One day I happened to mention the situation to a colleague who was a psychiatric-oncology nurse at a large military medical center. He was not at all surprised by my experience and explained:

> I've worked as a clinical specialist in psych-oncology for years, and I see patients frequently during the chemo experience. I talk with them about their pain and anxiety and fear of death, and about the stigma of their disease. They look forward to my visits. I'm a sounding board and a friend. But … once the chemotherapy is over and they've recovered, they don't want to know me anymore. If I see one of my former patients at a military function or an exercise, they will look away or walk right past me as if we had never met. At first it hurt but then I began to understand that I was so identified with their cancer experience that they had to forget me. I reminded them of their disease which they want to forget.

My and my colleague's patients needed, as Suzanne Gorden suggests, to "flee the memory" of our involvement in their lives; we had become anonymous.

In my two previous books, *Spirituality and Nursing: Standing on Holy Ground*[38] and *The Nurse's Calling: A Christian Spirituality of Caring for the Sick*,[39] I described nurses as "anonymous ministers." Some of the most significant and powerful interactions nurses have with their patients, some of their most important spiritual interventions, are never charted, never discussed, never reported, and never formally acknowledged by

supervisors or administrators. Yet these actions may be incredibly influ-
ential in the coping response and/or outcome of a patient's illness and
treatment. These unacknowledged and anonymous nursing acts are truly
courageous acts of love and caring; they are actions that connect the contemporary nurse to her historical prefigure, Veronica of Jerusalem.

A NURSES' WAY OF THE CROSS

As explained in the earlier discussion of Saint Veronica's "legend,"
many Christians' familiarity with Veronica's compassionate act, per-
formed for Jesus during his passion, is derived from their prayerful practice of the "Way of the Cross." Nurses, in the course of their profession,
may experience their own unique way of the Cross, through encountering
and embracing their patients' sufferings. These observations and interactions can be included in a nurse's prayer life through associating his or
her patients' agonies with those of Our Blessed Lord in meditations and
prayers that constitute a "Nurse's Way of the Cross."

1. Jesus Is Condemned to Die.

He's a fine young man, a boy really, only 16 when the symptoms
first start: the headaches, the dizziness, and the nausea. Not so bad, at
first; probably too many hours on the new computer he thinks, or maybe
just worry about those upcoming SATs. But then one morning he can't get
out of bed and the round of testing begins, and the surgery. An invasive
glioblastoma, the neurosurgeon said; we couldn't get it all. He is con-
demned to die, this innocent, whose only crime was choosing to embrace
his teenage life.

> *Dear Lord Jesus, who in your own innocence, was condemned to die*
> *for choosing to embrace our fragile world, help my patients to em-*
> *brace their physical condemnations. I get angry sometimes; it seems*
> *so unfair. I can't understand; I don't ask to. Only grant me the grace*
> *to cross over; to stand as your loving presence with those condemned*
> *to death from illness or disease.*

2. Jesus Takes Up His Cross.

"The breast cancer has spread to the lymph nodes," they tell the
young mother. There's a husband and two toddlers to think of; "we'll

begin an aggressive program of treatment" the oncology team advises. "We can't save your hair, not with this much chemotherapy," they admit, but "don't worry, the wigs they make these days are pretty good." "Mommy, Mommy, pick me up," the little ones cry in unison. "Mommy loves you so much," she replies, "but right now Mommy is sick. She has to rest. But don't ever forget: Mommy loves you!"

Blessed Lord Jesus, you took up such a heavy Cross for us. Help me to accept the crosses that sickness and disability impose. Taking up a cross is a fearful task but You, Dear Lord, blessed the action with Your love and compassion. Teach me to help my patients look to You for courage and strength as they struggle to take up their personal crosses.

3. Jesus Falls for the First Time.

Everything seems to be going well with the new therapeutic regimen. The brittle juvenile onset diabetes that has dominated his life for so many years is under control. The disease is a cross but it's become manageable, or so the young teacher thinks. All he wants is to enjoy the end of school party with his class of boisterous eighth graders. They don't understand his need for a delicate balance of exercise, diet, and medication. He wakes up that evening in the medical ICU; the hurt to his body is modest, the hurt to his spirit grievous.

Dearest Jesus, it's really hard to fall when you think that the path before you will be smooth. It hurts not only the body but also the heart. Help me to be there to catch my patients when they fall; help me especially to catch their spirits that I might lift them up to you.

4. Jesus Meets His Sorrowful Mother.

She's a small woman, with dark hair, no grey yet or at least she hides it well, and a kind and gentle smile; only her eyes reveal the terrible sadness in her heart. "This is my Mom" the young cancer patient says proudly. He has something called stage IV rhabdomyosarcoma; it's too horrible a label for a 21 year old, and he's in the advanced stages of the disease. The mother's courage is overwhelming. In his room she teases, cajoles, supports, and loves; she is his mother. In the hallway she dissolves into heart-wrenching sobs; she is his mother.

Blessed Lord, Your own beloved mother's heart was pierced by a cruel sword. Help me to minister to the mothers and fathers of my young patients. Teach me to touch their pain with gentleness, so that I may stand with them as a caring companion on their journeys of suffering. Help me, also, to be myself a "mother" to those for whom I care.

5. Simon of Cyrene Helps Jesus Carry His Cross.

Paul, the young unit clerk on the childrens' oncology ward is bald; I mean really bald, like the proverbial "billiard ball." I asked the staff about it. "Is he a chemo patient himself?" I wondered, or "Is shaving off all one's hair some kind of contemporary statement?" "Oh, it's definitely a statement," the nursing staff replied. "You see, Paul knows how hard it is for the children on chemotherapy to lose their hair; it's especially tough on the teens. So Paul decided to shave off his own hair so that the children won't feel alone. He did it as a sign of support." Amazing! this dear young Paul "of Cyrene."

Blessed Lord Jesus, the weight of your heavy Cross was lightened by the young, strong arms of Simon. Teach me, as a nurse, to use my arms and my heart to lighten the painful suffering of those I care for. Teach me to have the courage of Simon in the practice of my nursing.

6. Veronica Wipes the Face of Jesus.

They brought him into the ER on the rescue squad gurney; it took two paramedics to hold him down. He was fighting the IVs and the oxygen just as he'd always had to fight for his life. That's the way it is living on the mean city streets. When he relaxed a little, a nurse tenderly washed the blood and grit from his eyes and face. "God bless you," he breathed softly through bruised and swollen lips. And God did.

My dearest Lord, you know about struggling for life. You experienced human cruelty in the most devastating way; you were betrayed by those you came to save. We nurses have the precious gift of being able to comfort our patients as Veronica comforted you in your time of suffering. Teach me to honor and reverence the gift.

7. Jesus Falls for the Second Time.

This time he was "sure he could do it," the ragged, trembling ER patient tells his nurse. Alcohol has ruled his life for so very long. "No more," he had decided, "no more!" Now his eyes reflect the pain and the shame of a resolve shattered and broken. The weight of his addiction is so heavy. He has fallen once again; "yes, it happened before," he admits. But, he desperately struggles to rise again and regain his fragile foothold on life.

> *My Dear Lord Jesus, in your blessed humanity, you chose to experience the pain of a heavy Cross, and to embrace the shame of falling beneath its weight. Teach me to accept my own human weaknesses; and teach me never to judge the weaknesses of my patients when they fall.*

8. Jesus Comforts the Women of Jerusalem.

His wife and his mother and his sister were all in the room; they looked heartbroken. "Don't be so grim," he teased them with a twinkle in his eye. "I can beat this thing; that tumor's probably been growing for years. I've still got lots of time to get in your hair; you can't get rid of me yet!" He tried to sound gruff but his eyes were filled with love and care for his dear ones and their pain.

> *My Beloved Lord, you knew what lay ahead; you knew about the suffering and you knew about the shame. Yet, in your own terrible pain, you reached out and comforted the women who loved you. Help my patients to have the strength and the courage to comfort their loved ones; help me to lift them up to you in their sorrow that they also may be comforted.*

9. Jesus Falls for the Third Time.

This one was supposed to be the winner. Twice before a donated kidney had become available, but the match just wasn't there. This time it was, the surgeon said: "Well, maybe not perfect but good enough." And for a while the "good enough" seemed to hold. But then the rejection symptoms began; mild at first, but soon beyond all help. Despite the nephrology team's "full court press," she has to return to dialysis. It's a crushing fall.

> *My Lord Jesus, when you experienced that third painful fall it must have been devastating. Did you wonder if you could rise again and complete the awful journey? Help me to reach out to my patients when they fall. Help me to help them stand and embrace their journey of living.*

10. Jesus Is Stripped of His Garments.

They rushed him into the burn unit in the middle of the night. The fire had incinerated his small frame house in minutes; it stripped off 70 percent of his skin in the process. The pain was unbearable; it couldn't get much worse. He hadn't the strength to moan but his eyes told the tale. We did what we could.

> *Dear Lord Jesus, it's so hard to see patients hurting so much, especially when an illness or accident strips them of their human dignity. Help me to remember to always reverence the sacredness of human life.*

11. Jesus Is Nailed to the Cross.

This was the first time she would be attached to the hemodialysis machine. She had known it was coming; there was a history of polycystic kidneys. It was the loss of control that seemed the worst part. To be forced to sit, unmoving, while all of her blood is circulating through a monstrous machine. "I feel like I'm about to be nailed to a cross," she sighed.

> *Blessed Lord Jesus, it's so very hard to lose control; You know. Teach me to be gentle with my patients in their frustration; teach me to help them bear their losses with grace and with dignity.*

12. Jesus Dies on the Cross.

She was only 42 years old but had been on the ventilator for almost three weeks now. The battle with ALS (amyotrophic lateral sclerosis) was long and tortuous; she was more than ready, but the family hadn't been willing to let go. Finally, they said, "Enough, we can't watch her suffer anymore." Her family surrounded the bed; her physician was there, as were the primary care nurse, the hospital chaplain, and a young med student who had grown to love her. They "pulled the plug," but tenderly and with great sadness. They experienced the blessing of praying her into eternal life.

> *My dearest Jesus, you knew human death intimately; you who chose to experience the passage in its fullness because you loved so deeply. It's a frightening thing; this letting go of everyone and everything we know. But you taught us to know your Father in heaven. Help me to midwife my patients into His loving presence in eternity.*

13. Jesus Is Taken Down from the Cross.

He was a junior student nurse doing his first "clinical" when he pulled the "short straw." We need help with postmortem care they told him. He had cared for the patient just yesterday. Sweet little Mrs. O'Reilly was a fragile 93 year old; she had just succumbed to her most recent stroke. As the student gently washed the body of his patient, he thought: "This is someone's mother; this is someone's wife, this is someone's friend." This is Jesus.

Blessed Lord Jesus, teach me to see you in each patient I care for. It's hard to lose those who have touched our spirits. Help me to remember that they are now with you; that they are not lost to us, and that their memory and all they shared in life will live on in the hearts of those who loved them.

14. Jesus Is Placed in the Tomb.

I didn't want to go to the funeral. He was so young, only 26 years old. I had grown to love him during those last months of the toxoplasmosis battle; I wanted to remember him as strong and vital; the way he was when first we met. It was just too soon for a funeral. But he had asked for a celebration of his life. So, celebrate we did, through the tears and the laughter and the terrible ache that squeezed your heart like a tight steel band. It was just too soon!

You understand, dearest Lord Jesus. You were only 33 years old and it seemed just too soon for you also. But You, the Divine Son, knew that Your Father's time is not our time. And you embraced the tomb that we might celebrate your life forever. Teach us to treasure the magnificent gift that your death and entombment was for us: Jesus of Nazareth, who died and rose and became for all humanity, Jesus, the Christ.

15. Jesus Is Risen from the Dead.

The Mass of Christian Burial is over. The service had been poignant and healing; the sympathy of family and friends had been genuine and loving. But now the parents must go home, alone, to enter the barren house that once echoed with childhood laughter. The tomb is empty; how can they bear the loss? They hold each other gently and remember the words their pastor had quoted so tenderly from scripture: "I am the resurrection and the life; whoever believes in me even if he dies, will live; and everyone who lives and believes in me will never die" (John 11: 25). Their precious child now lives with the Lord; this is their consolation and their strength.

> *Dear Risen Lord Jesus, who promised life to all who believe in you, comfort those who mourn. Ease the grievous loss of loved ones with the gift of hope in a promise of eternal salvation. Grant the bereaved the blessing of your tender love in their time of sorrow and lead them, finally, to Your Sacred Heart, where alone they may find solace and peace.*

PRAYER AND A HEALING MINISTRY

The theme of this chapter has been the association between a nurse's Journey to Jerusalem and his or her healing ministry. Jerusalem, in the time of Jesus, was a place of suffering but it was also a "holy place";[40] and a "religious" place.[41] Jerusalem became, with Jesus' death and resurrection, a place of healing and of redemption. Each of the four evangelists, in describing Jesus' entry into Jerusalem, focused on a different dimension of his ministry. Matthew, who saw Jesus' donkey as a beast of burden emphasized the "humble" nature of his arrival;[42] Mark noted that Jesus' entry to the holy city fulfilled his "prophet-Savior" role;[43] Luke suggested that "riding on an ass was not so much an emphasis on humility as on peacefulness";[44] and John's gospel highlighted the fact that, although Jesus was victorious, he rode "not a stallion of war but the donkey of service."[45] Thus, four key characteristics of Jesus' healing ministry as reflected in the evangelists' descriptions of his final preparation to go to the Father, can be understood as humility, peace, service, and salvation. These concepts provide powerful guideposts to direct a nurse's healing ministry.

Humility

> *"And all of you, clothe yourselves with humility in your dealings with one another, for / 'God opposes the proud / but bestows favor on the humble.' So humble yourselves under the mighty hand of God, that he may exalt you in due time."*
>
> 1 Peter 5: 5

To approach a patient or family member from the perspective of a healing ministry or healing practice, a nurse needs to be possessed of the virtue of humility. Humility is described by William Shannon as "grounded in a deep awareness of our limitations and shortcomings in the presence of the Divine perfection."[46] Father Shannon also observes that humility is a central component of contemporary spirituality and is viewed "not as self deprecation but as self honesty."[47] He cites the writings of Thomas Merton who viewed "the humble person as one who can achieve great things for God and for others" because he does not live for himself alone.[48]

A few years ago I was principal investigator of a complex nursing study exploring physical, psychosocial, and spiritual coping in life threatening illness. To understand our patients' response to their disease trajectories, the study team asked a number of both structured and open-ended questions. Some of the items in our interviews were of a sensitive and personal nature, such as questions dealing with religious and spiritual beliefs, and supportive relationships.

Early on in the study, one of my most capable and compassionate psych-mental health nurse research team members expressed concern about the need for humility: "We really have to be humble to work with these patients," he said. "I didn't know how tough it would be to ask all those questions. I feel like I'm asking to be allowed to enter very private places in the patients' lives, and I have to approach it with a lot of gentleness and humility." In expanding on his thoughts, my research associate expressed some surprise at how deeply aware the work had made him of the nurse's need for humility: "I never really thought about it before," he said, "but the research made me realize the responsibility and the gift we have as nurses. It's humbling to realize that, and it makes you know that you have to approach your nursing with real humility."

A historical maxim that undergirds a nurse's need for humility is Florence Nightingale's classic comment: "And remember every nurse … must have a respect for her own calling, because God's precious gift of life is often literally placed in her hands."[49] Frequently, I believe that we nurses, and I surely put myself at the top of the list, lose sight of the immensity of our mission and ministry of caring for God's most fragile ones. Sometimes, in truth, we have the physical survival of a patient in our hands, for example during such a complex therapy as hemodialysis; other times we may have the opportunity to support a patient's emotional or spiritual well being, simply through our caring presence. Whatever our nursing ministry calls for, we must pray for the blessing of humility in all that we do; we must never forget that our work is guided by the hand of the Divine Physician who walks by our side and who carries us when our own steps falter. The gift of humility will help us to recognize and rejoice in the joy of being earthen vessels who hold a treasure within; a treasure which is the light of Jesus the Lord.

Peace

"Peace I leave with you; my peace I give to you."

John 14: 27

Peace or peacefulness, from a Christian perspective, is reflected in the New Testament accounts of Jesus greeting his disciples with the word *peace*. It is noted that in the Lord's "Hebraic understanding, this greeting of peace, of shalom, spoke to a fullness of peace and wholeness permeating every act of a person's life."[50] This is a peace which Jesus, himself, made possible through his passion and death.[51]

A competent and caring nurse brings peacefulness to a patient through a healing ministry of compassion and skill. With such an approach, trust is engendered in the nurse-patient relationship; this trust decreases anxiety on the part of the ill person and allows for a sense of peace, even in the midst of suffering and struggle.

In working with people coping with a life-threatening illness, one of the greatest gifts that a nurse can give is to help fearful patients make peace with the uncertainty of their futures. David was such a patient. Newly diagnosed with Burkitt's lymphoma, he had initially faced both anxiety and depression about his disease prognosis. After some days of prayer ministry carried out by both nurses and hospital chaplains, however, David was able to be at peace with his condition: "Well this is not what I had expected at this time in my life, but this is the Cross, the folly of the Cross they say, so I put it in the hands of the 'man upstairs.' I mean I'm really with Him and He's with me." David's final comment reflects his sense of peacefulness in the words: "You know God is going to be walking beside you."[52]

Service

"Whoever serves, let it be with the strength that God supplies, so that in all things God may be glorified through Jesus Christ."

1 Peter 4: 11

"The Son of Man did not come to be served but to serve and to give his life as a ransom for many."

Mark 10: 45

The word *service* is derived from the Greek verb *diakoneo* meaning "to serve"; thus, the title Deacon was applied to "the first followers of Jesus who cared for the sick and the infirm."[53] It is asserted that Jesus' act of washing his disciples' feet "dramatically portrays the model of service he suggests for his followers."[54]

The concept of service has been central to the profession of nursing since its inception. Virtually all of the early hospitals, and many facilities still today, have Departments of Nursing Service. The act of serving or caring for those who are ill or infirm is the heart of a nurse's healing ministry. As an educator and researcher, my own service rarely involves the "hands-on" care of the nurse practitioner, yet my spirit is continually drawn to such caregiving; I believe it's the same for all nurses whatever our administrative or academic responsibilities. We are, as a profession, most blessed that we have the opportunity to serve and to heal as Veronica. Our prayer must be that we always remember to see the beloved face of Jesus in those we serve and in those we care for in our healing ministry of nursing.

Salvation

Scripture passages in both the Old and the New Testaments are replete with references to salvation: "The LORD is my light and my salvation" (Psalm 27: 1); "Make haste to help me, / O LORD and my salvation" (Psalm 38: 23); "Only in God is my soul at rest; / from him comes my salvation" (Psalm 62: 2); and, "Therefore, I bear with everything for the sake of those who are chosen, so that they too may obtain the salvation that is in Christ Jesus" (2 Timothy 2: 10); "Consider the patience of our Lord as salvation" (2 Peter 3: 15); "Today salvation has come to this house ... for the Son of Man has come to seek and to save what was lost" (Luke 19: 9–10).

Salvation has been described by theologian Frances Schussler-Fiorenza as "a healing, a bringing to health, or a making whole or well."[55] Although the Christian image of salvation immediately brings to mind the redemptive act of love encompassed by the Passion and death of Jesus, this concept has meaning also for us, as nurses, in our daily practice of a healing ministry. The definition of salvation articulated by Schussler-

Fiorenza, which focuses on the concepts of "healing" or "making whole," provides nursing with a strong spiritual dimension that is linked to the salvation ministry of Jesus.

We nurses surely do not, I believe, think of ourselves as "saviors." Nonetheless most of us can recall instances both in our own practices and in those of our coworkers when a patient has described a nurse as one who "saved" his or her life, either literally or figuratively. Such a remark may relate to excellent physical care, or it may have to do with the compassionate and caring nature of the nurse-patient interactions. Nurses working with acutely ill patients may find their activities focused primarily on ministry that leads to physical healing. Those nurses who work in specialty areas such as hospice care, oncology, or gerontology, however, may have different goals. Although physical healing can be part of their desired nursing outcome, frequently an undergirding theme of practice is to assist patients in achieving a sense of wholeness or "making whole" in preparation for the transition to eternal life.

In the end, however, it is only through prayer that nurses will truly be able to undertake a healing ministry of caring which incorporates the gifts of humility, peace, service, and salvation. Such a ministry of nursing will, no doubt, include a Journey to Jerusalem for each individual practitioner. Nurses are blessed to be able to use their own wounds, incurred during this journey, to become superb "wounded healers." Nurses are blessed to have the opportunity to live out a daily ministry of healing, modeled by our Lord and Savior, the greatest healer of all. This is a blessing we must never take for granted; this is a blessing we must daily thank God for. This is the blessing of a healing ministry, supported and blessed by the healing ministry of Jesus of Nazareth, our Master Teacher and our Lord.

A NURSE'S PRAYER TO BECOME A HEALER

> *"Everyone in the crowd sought to touch him because power came forth from him and HEALED them all."*
>
> Luke 6: 19

O God, who heals our hurts and calms our fears with the passion of Your love, teach me to be a healer. Gift my nursing that it may be blessed with the soothing balm of a tender touch, the comforting peace of a caring spirit, and the healing grace of a loving heart. Help me to step out with the courage and compassion of the healer Veronica, as I tenderly minister to the ill and the infirm. May I never forget to see, in the countenance of each person I serve, the Blessed image of Your Divine Son. Amen.

8 ✣ The Art of Contemplative Caregiving

"Rising very early before dawn, he left and went off to a deserted place, where he prayed."

Mark 1: 35

CONTEMPLATIVE NURSING

Gentle God,
  You alone are the source of my strength
    and the center of my life.
  how I ache to live those words in
    my nursing.
  But I'm so fragile; so often I forget
    who You really are.
  I keep pretending that I am the source
    of my strength and the center of
    my life, instead of You.
  And then, on a bad day, it all starts
    unraveling.

  How can I nurse with gentleness and compassion
    in so challenging a health care
      system?
  There are so many complicated issues; they
    hinder my caregiving at every turn.
  Sometimes I wonder what it is that keeps
    me going.

  But, just when things seem darkest, a tiny
    glimmer of light appears.

Gnarled, arthritic fingers seek out my hand
and a small, frail voice whispers to my
   heart: "Thank you for being my nurse;
   God bless you!"

   And You do!

For, suddenly, in that fragile moment, I
  remember that You, my God, are ever
  with me;
    waiting with outstretched arms
    and loving embrace.

I remember that You use my hands to touch
  with Your tenderness those who are
   suffering and sorrowful.
  I remember that You use my eyes to look
   with Your reverence on those who are
   rejected and reviled.
   I remember that You use my heart to
   love with Your love those who are
   lonely and afraid.

I lay my head gently on Your shoulder and
  I bathe in Your nearness.
   "Don't be afraid,"
    You breathe the words into my
    soul,

      "For I am with you always.
      Hold tight to my hand
      and don't let go.
      I won't!"

And, now, I remember, again, Dear Lord,
  that You are indeed the source
   of my strength and
    the center of my life.

This is the reward of ministering to the
  sick in Your Name.

This is the joy of meeting Your Son
  in caring for the ill and the
    infirm.

This is the blessing of
  contemplative nursing.

  Teach me to live
      and
  to treasure
    the gift.

The day dawned clear and brisk that Christmas Eve, and my school of nursing's campus had been embellished with a brilliant coat of glistening frost. The scene was an elegant memento of a recent and unexpected East Coast snowfall. Our usually green lawns were carpeted in pristine blankets of white; the tree branches decorated with shimmering crystal ice ornaments. An etherial specter of enchanted winter wonderland now graced our usually busy and functional workplace.

I had stayed on campus that holiday to write, and thus had the gift of attending a prayerful Midnight Mass at the church adjacent to our university; the worship space was filled to overflowing with those who had come to celebrate the feast of the Birth of Jesus. The service provided a wonderful experience of communal Christian prayer.

As I stepped out of the church, after Mass, I was suffused with the warm glow of the joyful celebration: the sacred liturgy, the inspiring music, and the shared worship with the assembled community of Christians. But my breath was almost taken away when I gazed at the beautiful winter scene before me. As I crossed the snow-covered campus on the way to my room, I couldn't help but reflect on the goodness of God who so beautifies our earth that we might delight in His creation. The natural world provides an exquisite setting for prayerful meditation on the greatness of our God; who must you be, O Lord of life, who created all of this? As the Psalmist teaches: "Great is the Lord and worthy to be praised; God's grandeur is beyond understanding" (Psalm 145: 3).

Because the hour was late and because I had a number of activities planned for Christmas morning, I had anticipated going straight to bed after the midnight service. As I entered my residence hall, however, I was intuitively drawn to a small university chapel where I knew that Jesus was alone and waiting, always waiting, for us to come to Him. The chapel was quiet, and dark and cold, a stark contrast to the bustling and magnificently decorated church I had just left. Only a sanctuary lamp burned reverently on the altar, an ever faithful witness to the presence of He who is the light of the world. Almost unconsciously I sank to my knees before the One who is the source of my strength and the center of my life; I was embraced by His love. Our quiet hour of being together that Christmas night was one of the most wonderful presents I have ever received from the Lord; I thank Him for it to this day. Prayer is indeed God's greatest gift to us; and it must be treasured beyond all others.

BEGINNING TO PRAY: FIVE STEPS IN PREPARATION FOR PRAYER

As I was reflecting on the narrative in the previous section, I realized that in that one evening I had experienced myriad kinds of prayer. The formal Christmas service encompassed communal worship that included four usually identified types of prayer: prayer of petition, prayer of thanksgiving, prayer of adoration, and prayer of confession or repentance. On my walk across the campus, I engaged in personal meditation on the goodness of God in relating to the beauty of the winter scene before me. And finally, during the hour of solitary prayer in my residence hall chapel, I was graced with a time of contemplation; the joy of simply being with the Lord and experiencing His love.

In the rest of this chapter, these and other kinds of prayer are discussed in terms of their relevance for those of us who care for the sick. It's important to remember, however, as discussed in the previous chapters, that one may not always have an emotionally positive response to prayer. The Lord sometimes gives us joy and satisfaction in prayer as a gift; our feelings, nonetheless, have nothing at all to do with the validity or the goodness or worthiness of our prayer. The simple act of coming before the Lord in prayer, in whatever way we are able at a particular time, is a spiritual activity worthy of His blessing.

I have written a lot, in earlier chapters, about the history of prayer in nursing, the prayer and nurse-patient relationships, the need for prayer in nursing, and even the difficulties one might experience such as distraction and dryness in prayer. But how does one begin to pray, or how can one strengthen or improve one's current prayer life? What should one say in prayer? These are questions frequently asked by those who are serious about developing a relationship with the Lord.

One of my favorite scholars of prayer, Jesuit William Barry, advises that while the specific how and where of prayer may vary with individuals, we have to recognize that "quality relationships need quality time to develop."[1] Certainly it is appropriate and advisable to whisper a quick prayer on the run if that is all the time you have at the moment; however, longer prayer times will be needed later in the process of developing a relationship with the Lord. Another Jesuit, Thomas Green, suggests that establishing a prayer relationship with God requires a time of "courtship"; part of that courtship is getting to know who God is. This can be accomplished by such activities as meditating on God's creation or on Scripture; the latter is important especially as one attempts to learn the life and the way of Jesus.[2] To answer the question "What should we say when we pray?" Peter Kreeft addresses the four themes of prayer: repentance, adoration, petition and thanksgiving as acts of love: repentance, or saying "I'm sorry," is faithful love asking for forgiveness; adoration is a statement of one's deepest love and respect; petition is trusting love asking for something for ourselves or for others; and thanksgiving is the giving back of love in gratitude for gifts given to us.[3] The words we use in our prayers of repentance, adoration, petition, and thanksgiving will be our own; that is the creativity of our prayer as in any conversation between people who are in love.

Another frequently asked question about prayer is "are there techniques or methods of prayer one should use?" I feel ambivalent about addressing the idea of "methods" of prayer because personal prayer may vary greatly depending upon an individual's personality, needs, experience, and religious tradition. One spiritual writer suggests that love is "too simple, too free and too great" for techniques or methods;[4] another feels that we do need a few methods that "fit us the best" but that we should avoid becoming overburdened by too many techniques of prayer.[5] I personally believe that where one is in the process of developing his or her relationship with the Lord will dictate which, if any, methods will be helpful; the methods used may also change across one's lifetime as life stages and life demands change.

Having said all that, I have to admit that I am still asked by colleagues to identify some steps to take in preparing oneself for a time of prayer. Although I am loathe to interfere with the action of the Holy Spirit, perhaps a few of the practical steps I personally have used might be helpful. *First*, I try to block out some uninterrupted time for prayer; this block of time may be in the morning, the evening, or any time in between, when I think I might be able to escape the telephone, email, or face-to-face interactions with others besides the Lord. He is my best friend, after all, and surely deserves my full attention when we are together. *Second*, I look for a place to pray that will be both quiet and relatively comfortable. As much as I love the one-hundred-year-old chapel in the residence where I live, I really find it difficult to pray when the temperature soars over 100 degrees in the hot and humid Washington, D.C., summers. (There was no air-conditioning in the nineteenth century!) While I usually prefer to pray in a chapel or church, I have often found my own room to be a wonderfully peaceful setting for prayer. Some things that help me settle down in this space, after a busy day, are the lighting of a candle and/or playing religious music softly; I also like sitting on the floor or using a small prayer bench to place my body in a prayerful attitude. Weather permitting, the outdoors can also provide a magnificent natural prayer environment; some days I just like to go for a walk with the Lord.

A *third* step to beginning a time of prayer, which I have discussed earlier, might be to open the Bible to a favorite passage; this step helps orient one's mind away from the problems of the day, or perhaps even toward the problems of the day, but in the light of God's love and guidance rather than one's own insights. If I am really worried about something, a passage from one of the psalms of God's protecton is a powerful reminder of the Lord's care, for example: "You know me when I sit and stand; you understand my thoughts from afar ... behind and before you encircle me and rest your hand upon me" (Psalm 139, v.1; 5); or "God will not allow your foot to slip; your guardian does not sleep ... the Lord will guard your coming and going both now and forever" (Psalm 121, v.3; 8).

A *fourth* step in preparation for prayer is to become interiorly quiet before the Lord. This step may be the most difficult in preparing for a time of prayer; at least, it can be for me. I sometimes feel like I have spent the first half or even three quarters of the time I had allotted for prayer trying to clear my mind, to let go of the many "important" thoughts running around in my head, either from the day that has just ended or regarding the day that is about to begin. I have to keep reminding myself that the most "important" thing I can do in prayer is just be present to the Lord; unfortunately, I am a very slow learner.

And then, after the first four steps have been taken, the most important step in beginning to pray is, of course, to listen. Surely it is a good thing to ask that our needs be met, to tell the Lord about our concerns for ourselves and for our loved ones, but the ultimate goal of a developing prayer life is to learn to listen to the Lord. The Holy Spirit's whisperings and His guidance can only be heard in the silence of a quiet soul, in the silence of an undistracted mind, and in the silence of an undivided heart. This focus is what we must attempt to bring to our times of prayer: a mind and a spirit totally focused on the One who is the center of our lives and the source of our strength, and a heart filled with love for Him, who alone can ease the yearning described so poignantly by Augustine: "Our hearts are restless, O Lord, until they rest in Thee."

For those of us who have busy schedules most days of the week, a structured morning prayer can be very helpful in setting a tone for the day. I find it important to attend Mass and pray the morning prayer of the Divine Office each day; that arrangement may not work for others depending upon religious tradition, work schedule, or prayer needs. I do feel, however, that to plan on some time for prayer on arising, even if abbreviated, is both necessary and comforting for those of us who care for the sick (or who teach or supervise those who minister to the ill). It's also very important for developing our relationship with God. Imagine if, in your household, you got up in the morning, showered, dressed, had your coffee or filled a cup to take in the car, and rushed out the front door without even saying "good morning" to the people with whom you live. You may just give your loved ones a quick "good morning" greeting or a hug; the point is that you have done something to make a connection. You have acknowledged, even if briefly, the love that exists between you and the significant others in your life; should it not be the same with the one who is the greatest love of our lives?

I think for us nurses it is often not so difficult beginning to pray privately; we have much to pray about. But for myself, and students and colleagues have also admitted to this, there can be a shyness about praying aloud with others or about leading a group in prayer. One of my nurse practitioner students, a deeply spiritual woman, told me that it took some degree of courage to begin to pray with her chemotherapy patients; she now does it regularly, for those patients who wish her to pray with them, but she admits that she is still somewhat shy about initiating the prayers.

We must, however, learn to take the risk. A number of years ago, when I was a new teacher, I initiated the routine of beginning all my nursing classes with a prayer. I reasoned that it would be good for the students; truth be told, I think that I needed the prayers more than the students did. At any rate, that first semester I have to admit to having had no little anxiety about the practice. My rather large class was composed of nursing students from a variety of age categories, racial and ethnic backgrounds, and religious traditions. Although I tried to choose the prayers and meditations carefully, my insecurity caused me to be quite sensitive to students' responses. Overall, the reactions were very positive. Often, after class, students would comment on the day's prayer; some even asked for copies for themselves.

In one of the classes, however, I became aware of a seeming non-response from one of my best and brightest students. She was a lovely young woman who always sat near the front of the classroom. When I began a prayer, she would lower her eyes and look very serious; she never seemed to acknowledge any reaction regarding the meaningfulness of a prayer, as did many others in the group. I really began to worry that perhaps my prayers were "turning her off."

One day our class was delayed in getting started; some of the early arriving students had initiated questions about an upcoming assignment. I spent about 10 minutes answering questions and clarifying points as the class gathered; the young woman about whom I had been concerned came late, whispering an apology about the "terrible traffic." When all of the group were present, I began to barrel into the day's lecture; suddenly, I noticed a hand waving at me from the middle of the classroom. When I acknowledged the student, she said: "Sister, aren't we going to pray today?" In the throes of our discussion, I had totally forgotten the opening prayer. The next exclamation was from my late student. She said: "Oh I'm so glad we haven't prayed yet! All I could think of while I was stuck in traffic was 'I'm going to miss our prayer'"; she added, "I really look forward to it!"

And I had almost stopped praying because, in my shyness and insecurity, I was so worried about offending this student. We need to risk.

CONTEMPLATIVE PRAYER IN NURSING

From a nonreligious perspective, the verb *contemplate* simply means to ponder or to think seriously about a subject. The religious connotation is similar, although the concept of contemplation generally is used to describe a particular kind of prayerful reflection. The following section will very briefly explore the methods or techniques of contemplative or mental prayer identified as meditation (including *Lectio Divina*); centering prayer, and contemplation.

Meditation

In his *Primer on Prayer*, Bartholomew O'Brien makes a straightforward distinction between meditation and contemplation. "To think only," he asserts, "is that form of mental prayer called meditation; to love only is that form of mental prayer called contemplation."[6] Meditation is sometimes viewed as a preparation for contemplation, of listening to and loving the Lord, but it is also an end itself when practiced as a prayerful discipline.[7] Meditation, or thinking about some spiritual matter, has the capacity to open our hearts to the divinity of the present moment;[8] the truth upon which one is meditating may pass from the mind into the heart, thus evoking a "loving, faith filled response" in the person praying.[9]

Although there are surely no perfect circumstances to facilitate meditation, Michael Casey offers some possible aids to meditation which include a regular time, good physical health, emotional equilibrium, social harmony, winding down, a suitable place, good posture, and attention to breathing.[10] These suggestions reflect the ideal, however, and are not absolutely necessary conditions for meditation. For example, "good physical health" surely does not mean that a person with either acute or chronic health problems cannot meditate. But if one was dealing with a nasty case of the flu, for example, one might take appropriate medications, force fluids, and get some rest before beginning a period of meditation.

Meditation is not always easy as it "engages every part of us: our mind, our emotions, our imagination, our creativity and, supremely, our will."[11] These criteria, I believe, reflect the signs of true meditative prayer. It can be very easy, for me at least, to slip from meditation to daydreaming or distraction if I do not really try to engage my mind, my heart, my imagination, and especially my will in pondering a spiritual thought.

Topics for prayerful meditation may be derived from many sources. I gave an example earlier of thinking about God's goodness when witnessing the beauty of nature; a similar reflection about the Lord may come from seeing the beauty and the courage in people, or in the complex functioning of the world around us. I remember a priest retreat master once advising a group of nurses I was with that whenever we saw a beautiful sunset, or the gentleness of a small animal, or the unconditional love of a young child, we should immediately refer that experience to God and say in meditative prayer: "Who must you be who created this from nothing?" I believe we can find that same kind of reference to the greatness and the goodness of God in our nursing practice, for example in such behaviors as the tender care of a sick child's parent; the selfless courage of a terminally ill teen, or the gentle compassion of a loving caregiver.

Lectio Divina

A unique and specific form of meditation upon Holy Scripture, the word of God, was labeled by the early monastics as *Lectio Divina* or holy reading; it is a practice now being taken up by many of today's lay Christians, as well as by contemporary monastic men and women. Carmelite Jean-Marie Howe suggests that *lectio* is for some people "an untapped source of spiritual wealth" because she notes, *lectio* encompasses not just holy reading but prayer and meditation as well. "We pass from one phase or aspect to the next quite naturally, without strenuous effort ... under the influence of the Spirit."[12] *Lectio* is "not a method of prayer," asserts Thelma Hall, "but rather parallels that human experience of the development of a deeply loving interpersonal relationship" with God;[13] in *lectio* God directly "addresses each person individually."[14]

Trappist Abbot Basil Pennington describes the method of *Lectio Divina* as consisting of three steps: one comes into the presence of God with the assistance of the Holy Spirit, listening occurs through reading of the sacred text, and a word or phrase is adopted for meditation and prayerful response.[15] How precisely, in terms of time and place, *Lectio Divina* is practiced varies with individuals and in different settings such as in a monastery or in one's home. The basic point of the practice, wherever carried out, is that one meditates slowly on the Word of God, listens for a message through the inspiration of the Holy Spirit, and responds prayerfully in gratitude. Often the message of a morning *lectio* meditation will provide sustaining spiritual guidance throughout one's day.

Nurses who begin their workdays in the early morning may not have time for a full *lectio* meditation. However, even a brief reading from one of the Psalms or a passage from the New Testament can provide a nurse with a spiritual thought that will help keep him or her connected to God throughout the day's nursing activities.

Centering Prayer

Centering prayer, another method of mental prayer, is described by one of its earliest proponents, Trappist Thomas Keating, as "a method designed to facilitate the development of contemplative prayer."[16] Keating outlines the method as consisting of choosing a sacred word or thought symbolic of God and his activity in one's life, settling quietly to absorb the chosen symbol and God's presence within, returning immediately to the symbol if other thoughts occur, avoiding any analysis of wayward thoughts or feelings, and remaining in silence for a few minutes at the end of the centering prayer time.[17] Essentially, centering prayer is designed to move one from a more active kind of verbal or meditative prayer to a more receptive stance of openness to or resting in God's love and care.

For nurses, centering prayer is a prayerful activity that most probably will need to be done after work hours, when some leisure time is available. The method allows time and space for the person praying to put aside the cares and worries of the day and rest in the Lord. Actually, this kind of prayer might provide a wonderful transition from a day of formal nursing activities to an informal evening of household chores or recreation.

Contemplation

The term *contemplation* has been and still is assigned various meanings from a spiritual or religious perspective. Basic to the concept, however, is the fact that contemplation has to do with meditating on the presence of God understood "not by thought but by love."[18] To highlight this distinction, Francis De Sales once commented that meditation was the "mother of love" and contemplation was the "daughter of love."[19] Our thoughts in meditation can draw us to the love of God; the result is an experience of that love in contemplation.

Spiritual writers describe a number of understandings of contemplation: Brother Roger of Taize notes poignantly that contemplation is the "attitude in which our whole being is totally seized by the wonder of a presence ... by the reality of the love of God";[20] Thomas Keating asserts that contemplation takes us to the point of "communing beyond words, thoughts and feelings ... to the gifts of the Holy Spirit as the source of one's prayer";[21] and Morton Kelsey suggests that in contemplation we simply open ourselves to God; "we listen and behold."[22] In a similar vein, Duncan Basil observes poetically that "gazing in contemplation is enough. Friends are finding one another and becoming 'we' in the manner of lovers";[23] and Thelma Hall points out that contemplation is not some kind of reward or mark of singular virtue, it is simply the effect "of being literally 'in love with God' at the deepest level of the relationship with Him for which we are created."[24] In sum, the goal of contemplation is to be united with God.[25]

Many people are afraid of the concept of contemplation as it might seem to be a practice reserved for those who reside in monasteries or cloistered convents; considering contemplation, as just described, may evoke a sense of mistrust that one might not be called to such an intense relationship with the Lord.[26] If, however, we accept the goal of contemplation as union with God, surely all of us are called to contemplation and to a contemplative lifestyle. As noted in a contemporary exploration of the vocation of the lay contemplative: "Contemplation in the present era is conceived both as a specific practice of nondiscursive interior prayer and, more broadly, as an approach to life born out of a cultivated contemplative attitude."[27] An important point to remember is that the call to contemplative prayer, to a contemplative lifestyle, may differ greatly for individuals. Some may be called upon by the Lord to make more radical life changes; for others "a gentler adjustment may be asked … a contemplative life does not necessarily look the same in all persons."[28]

Contemplative caregiving may also not necessarily look the same for all nurses. The times, the places, the experiences of contemplative prayer, from which our contemplative caregiving is derived, are usually hidden, at least for those of us not living in convents or monasteries. Our meetings with the Lord are private and personal like the solitary trysts of lovers whose only desire is to be alone with each other. Our contemplative caregiving, as suggested in this chapter's opening meditation, is also hidden, manifested only by the tenderness, the reverence, and the love which emanate from ministering to the sick in His Name.

PRAYER AND SPIRITUAL READING

As discussed in Chapter 3, the most meaningful and important spiritual reading one may undertake to support a prayer life is that of Holy Scripture, the inspired Word of God. However, the spiritual writings of both early and later followers of the Gospel of Jesus can provide supplemental support and inspiration for the development of one's relationship with God. Spiritual reading, asserts authors Jacqueline Bergan and Marie Schwan, is "always enriching" to one's prayer life. They suggest the following process for spiritual reading: "Read slowly, pausing periodically to allow the words and phrases to enter within you. When a thought resonates deeply, stay with it, allowing the fullness of it to penetrate your being."[29]

There are magnificent Christian mystics, martyrs, and theologians whose writings, ranging from the classics of old to contemporary spiritual works, can be particularly helpful to nurses. The following suggestions may provide some guidance for a nurse seeking to begin or to flesh out his or her spiritual reading bookshelf.

Pre-Twentieth-Century Mystics, Martyrs, and Theologians

Hildegard of Bingen. Hildegard was a twelfth-century German mystic and Benedictine Abbess who was noted for her skill in caring for the sick; she has been described as both a physician and a nurse, having cared extensively for the sick monks in her Disibodenburg Abbey infirmary. The ill and infirm also came to the monastery from afar to consult Hildegard's healing powers. Hildegard wrote a number of books, one of which, *Liber Composite Medicinae*, dealt with diagnosing and treating illness and disease (see B. Lachman, *The Journal of Hildegard of Bingen*, 1998).

Francis of Assisi. Francis, as well as being a great thirteenth-century Italian saint and founder of the Franciscan order, was unfailing in his care for the sick and disabled, especially people suffering from the most stigmatized disease of his era, leprosy. Francis' loving ministry to lepers serves as a model for contemporary caregiving for those living with HIV and AIDS. (There are a plethora of biographies of Francis; one example is: O. Englebert, *St. Francis of Assisi*, 1982.)

Elizabeth of Hungary. Saint Elizabeth is described as a "patroness of nursing" because of her great dedication to care for the sick poor in the early 1200s. Although raised as a princess in Hungary, both prior to and following the untimely death of her husband, Elizabeth nursed the disenfranchised ill and disabled with her own hands, even bringing them home to her bed if need be. She established several hospitals and hospices and died at the young age of 24 (see E.R. Obbard, *Poverty My Riches: A Study of St. Elizabeth of Hungary 1207–1231*, 1999).

Mechtild of Magdeburg. Mechtild was a renowned mid-thirteenth century German mystic who spent most of her adult life in a community of "Beguines," a group of women who, though not formally vowed, dedicated their lives to prayer and service to the poor and the sick. Mechtild was hailed as a great spiritual director and was the author of a spiritual treatise *The Overflowing Light of the Godhead* (see S. Woodruff, *Meditations with Mechtild of Magdeburg*, 1996).

Julian of Norwich. Julian (sometimes called Juliana) was an English woman mystic whose life spanned the thirteenth and fourteenth centuries; she lived as an anchoress in a small cell next to St. Julian's church in Norwich. (Her given name is unknown; hence the title Julian of Norwich.) One of her greatest contributions to the literature of the era, focusing on holiness of life, was *The Showings of Julian of Norwich*. She is perhaps best known by contemporary readers for her motto: "All shall be well, all shall be well, and all manner of things shall be well" (see J. Walsh, *Julian of Norwich: Showings*, 1978).

Catherine of Siena (Patroness of Nursing). Catherine of Siena was a fourteenth-century Dominican tertiary who spent many hours caring for the sick poor during the Black Plague epidemic in Europe. Catherine was a mystic, with a brilliant mind, and an intense relationship with the Lord. On one occasion Jesus is said to have given her a ring as a sign of her status as His mystical spouse (see A.P. Baldwin, *Catherine of Siena: A Biography*, 1987).

The Cloud of Unknowing. This book is a spiritual classic written by an unknown English mystic who lived during the fourteenth century. The theme of the *Cloud of Unknowing* is that we cannot, with our finite minds, ever really know who God is. God is beyond our understanding and there exists a "cloud of unknowing" between humanity and the Divine. The anonymous author does, however, point out that God can, to a degree, be known through loving contemplative prayer that may "pierce" the cloud. (There are a variety of editions of The Cloud with introduction and commentary; one example, for a new reader of the work, is a small volume entitled *Where Only Love Can Go: A Journey of the Soul into the Cloud of Unknowing*, J. Kirwin, 1996.)

Teresa of Avila. Teresa of Avila was a sixteenth-century Spanish Carmelite mystic who achieved notable reform of Carmelite women's religious communities. She is famous for expressions such as "Let nothing disturb you, nothing dismay you, all things are passing, God never changes." Teresa is known to have had a very strong personality and a secure relationship with the Lord. On one occasion, when Teresa was unhappy with something that happened to her, she believed that she heard God say: "This is how I treat my friends." Teresa's petulant response was, "It is no wonder then Lord, that you have so few of them" (see C. Medwick, *Teresa of Avila: The Progress of a Soul*, 1999).

John of the Cross. John of the Cross was also a sixteenth-century Spanish Carmelite mystic, and although some years younger, a contemporary and friend of Teresa of Avila. John also sought to reform his community but suffered greatly during the Inquisition. His classic contributions to the literature include *The Ascent of Mt. Carmel* and *The Dark Night of the Soul* (see *The Collected Works of Saint John of the Cross*, 1991).

Francis De Sales. Francis De Sales was a late sixteenth- and early seventeenth-century French Bishop and spiritual leader who preached a message of love and spiritual friendship, accessible to all. Together with Jeanne De Chantal, he founded a women's religious community, the Order of the Visitation, whose original purpose was to visit and care for the sick poor. De Sales' most important written contribution is his book,

An Introduction to the Devout Life, which can be useful for people in any state in life, seeking a spiritual path to God (see J.F. Power (ed.), *Francis De Sales: Finding God Wherever You Are,* 1996).

Vincent de Paul. Vincent de Paul, the great seventeenth-century saint, who loved and ministered to the poor in France, founded the Vincentian family, cofounding with Louise de Marillac a women's religious community, the Daughters of Charity. One of the Daughters' primary ministries was, and still is, to care for the sick poor in hospitals and in their homes. Vincent's image for the Daughters was unique, for his era, in his conceptualization that the Sisters not remain enclosed in a cloistered environment. A famous maxim, attributed to Saint Vincent, notes: "Your convent will be the houses of the Sick ... your cloister, the streets of the city" (see books by R.P. Maloney, *The Way of Vincent de Paul,* 1992, and *He Hears the Cry of the Poor: On the Spirituality of Vincent de Paul,* 1995).

Brother Lawrence of the Resurrection. Brother Lawrence, a seventeenth-century French Carmelite lay brother, is sometimes referred to as the "saint of the kitchen." He was for many years the monastery cook, yet he was recognized for his deep spirituality and wisdom. Brother Lawrence felt that all tasks, however simple, should be considered holy and provide opportunities for prayer and for developing our relationship with God. His spiritual maxims and conversations were published, after his death, in a small work called *The Practice of the Presence of God* (see C. De Meester, *The Practice of the Presence of God* [Critical Edition], 1994).

Damien of Molokai. As a young man, Father Damien De Veuster, a Belgian priest, requested to be assigned to the Hawaiian leper colony of Molokai. His mission was to provide love and care for those who had been forced to live out their days in illness and abandonment on the lonely island. Father Damien improved both medical and spiritual care for his congregation on Molokai in the later nineteenth century; he cared for many patients with his own hands, never concerned about contagion. A well-known anecdote about Father Damien relates that one morning, during a sermon at Mass, Damien announced that he himself had contracted the dreaded disease by simply using the expression: "We lepers!" (see G. Dans, *Holy Man: Father Damien of Molokai,* 1989).

Therese of Lisieux. The life of Saint Therese, nineteenth-century Carmelite mystic and "little flower" of Jesus, as she liked to call herself, is well known to many of us. Her "little way" of simplicity, and of seeing God's will in all aspects of our life, can provide helpful guides for an individual's personal spiritual journey. Recently, the plethora of literature about her life has increased. A classic work, nevertheless, remains her own autobiography, published after her death (see J. Beevers, trans., *The Autobiography of Saint Therese of Lisieux: The Story of a Soul*, 1987).

Twentieth- and Twenty-First-Century Spiritual Writers

There is, of course, a multiplicity of inspiring Christian spiritual writers from both the twentieth and the present century. Individual interest will direct which authors provide the best guidance for facilitating a nurse's prayer life. The spirituality of a few well-known authors (and some of their classic works) which might be helpful include *Henri Nouwen* (*Adam: God's Beloved*, 1997; *Can You Drink This Cup*, 1996; *The Genesse Diary: Report from a Trappist Monastery*, 1981; *The Road to Daybreak: A Spiritual Journey*, 1990; and *The Wounded Healer*, 1979); *Jean Vanier* (*An Ark for the Poor: The Story of L'Arche*, 1995; *Becoming Human*, 1999); *Richard Foster* (*Celebration of Discipline: The Path to Spiritual Growth*, 1988; *Prayer: Finding the Heart's True Home*, 1992); *Adrian Van Kaam* (*Becoming Jesus: The Diary of a Soul Touched by God*, 1998; *Spirituality and the Gentle Life*, 1974); *Hannah Hurnard* (*Hinds' Feet on High Places*, 1975); *Roger of Taize* (*His Love Is a Fire*, 1990; *No Greater Love*, 1991; *The Wonder of Love: A Letter from Brother Roger of Taize*, 1996); *Joan Chittister* (*The Rule of Benedict: Insight for the Ages*, 1998; *Wisdom Distilled from the Daily*, 1991); and *Mother Teresa* (*The Blessings of Love*, 1996; *Loving Jesus*, 1991; *No Greater Love*, 1997).

These lists are by no means exhaustive. There are many fine works by other spiritual writers, both early and more recent, which can be found in contemporary Christian bookstores and libraries.

JOURNALING

Journaling, or writing out a narrative of one's ideas, reflections, experiences, dreams or plans may take a number of forms. Some people like to document their thoughts in an actual "journal" or notebook of some type; others prefer to keep a running description of ideas on their PCs, or even on a cassette tape. Journaling may be done as often or as infrequently as the person journaling finds comfortable and satisfying. Each year, in the "spirituality and nursing" course I teach, I ask my students to keep a journal—for their benefit, not for a grade. In fact, I tell them that, if they prefer, I will not read their thoughts to preserve their privacy. This past year all of the students in the class purchased small personal journals, with bright attractive covers, to document their reflections and spiritual experiences. On the last day of class, in an informal "retreat" setting, the students chose to share portions of their journals with class-mates; most of us had tears in our eyes as we listened to the beautiful and poignant thoughts and experiences of those with whom we had spent the past class semester.

Not all nurses will choose to engage in journaling; for some it may seem like an added task rather than a prayerful activity. For others, how-ever, journaling can provide support for a developing prayer life, as well as serve as an outlet for personal concerns or stressors. Pierre Wolff, in his book on prayer, raises the question "Do I have to keep a journal?" His response, as my own, is essentially, it's up to you. An advantage, Wolff points out, is that keeping a journal about our prayer life will help us remember the things that were important in our spiritual journey. If one chooses to journal, Wolff suggests three point of focus for notes: "What has touched me?" "How much was I touched?" and "Why was I touched?"[30]

Journaling is sometimes described as "meditative writing" in the sense that "spirit and body cooperate to release our true selves."[31] An ex-citing thing about journaling, for me, is that I never know exactly what the end result will be when I begin to write. As Joseph Schmidt puts it: "When we take pen in hand, we grasp a door handle and begin to open areas of our life history and present awareness that are deeper than we had imag-ined."[32] Journaling can also be a prayerful experience in itself; God's grace may be channeled through the experience of writing.[33]

BECOMING A MYSTIC

As I mentioned earlier, during my theology studies I enrolled in a class on "The Mystics." The course immediately preceding "The Mystics" in our assigned classroom was a seminar on Canon Law. Being lawyers, the group always tended to run overtime, thus leaving the Mystics class waiting outside. Of course this gave my classmates and I the perfect open-ing to harass the canon lawyers for intruding on our time. They, in turn, informed us that it was altogether appropriate that the Mystics wait humbly in the hallway until the canon lawyers had finished their impor-tant deliberations.

It's fun being a student; there is, however, a point to my sharing the levity of the above interaction between student canon lawyers and student mystics. Those who have been described, historically, as mystics, although now perhaps well known to us, were during their lifetimes often humble and unassuming people. Therese of Lisieux immediately comes to mind. While we now recognize her as a saint and a doctor of the Church, she was in her era simply a relatively uneducated young Carmelite nun who died at the age of 24. Therese would, I'm sure, have been completely comfortable "waiting humbly in a hallway."

So, what does it mean to be a mystic, and are all of us called to a degree of mysticism in our lives? Mysticism is defined by Carmelite John Welch as "a loving knowledge of God which is born in a personal encounter" and, which results in "a way of life which is built upon one's direct experience of God."[34] He adds, "Today, mysticism ... is viewed as a common and normal activity, although often implicit, in the lives of all Christians."[35] Benedictine James Wiseman asserts that an "attitude of deep reverence toward God and one's fellow human beings is ... a fundamental sign of genuine mysticism."[36]

In previous writing I suggested that there was indeed a degree of "mysticism" in everyday nursing;[37] my analogy was based on the perspective of distinguished theologian Karl Rahner who believed that each of us is called to be "at least an anonymous mystic."[38] Rahner contended that even everyday life could be holy. "Wherever there is radical self-forgetting for the sake of the other ... there is ... the mysticism of everyday life."[39] Karl Rahner's understanding of mysticism surely supports the appropriateness of the call of every nurse to becoming a mystic.

In her book *Finding The Mystic Within You*, lay Carmelite Peggy Wilkenson cites the spiritual maxim: "Pray as you can, not as you ought."[40] I think that is a very comforting and realistic guideline for nurses seeking to find the "mystic within." It seems like I have been saying this over and over, but just as there are many ways to pray verbally and to meditate, there is also a variety of ways to encounter the Divine, to experience God and seek His direction in our lives. Sometimes I have a very prayerful experience of listening to the Lord in a chapel or a church; sometimes it happens during a long quiet walk; sometimes, in autumn, when I'm just sitting outdoors and watching the leaves surrender their lives so that new growth can blossom forth the following spring; and sometimes, in the spring, through delighting in the warmth of the sun and the beauty of the emerging landscape.

In our nursing, we have so many opportunities to encounter the Divine in the continuous cycles of death and birth, of illness and recovery, of suffering and healing. There is indeed, as Karl Rahner would say of life, a mysticism in our everyday nursing. And it is in reflecting on the experiences of everyday nursing, in prayer, that we will embrace that mysticism, that we will be able to find "the mystic within" our own spirits.

CONTEMPLATIVE CAREGIVING: THE NURSE WITH THE ALABASTER JAR

"O God, you are my God whom I seek; for you my flesh pines and my soul thirsts / like the earth, parched, lifeless and without water."
                                                      Psalm 63, 2–3

I used to long to run off to a monastery; to go to a solitary mountaintop to pray, to find holiness. I wanted to finish up, as quickly as possible, the nitty-gritty aspects of my daily responsibilities so that I could go on to greater things, to become a contemplative. And in truth, I still do long for that sometimes. But I realized one day that, in fact, the "seeds" of a contemplative soul need to be "watered" in the very mundane experiences of the everyday life that I wanted to escape. The problem is that it's not easy to be a contemplative, to practice contemplative caring, outside the structure of a monastic rule and lifestyle.

In discussing the "formation of the everyday contemplative," however, Stephen Hatch offers some practices that an aspiring contemplative might adopt: the regular practice of contemplative prayer, scheduled solitude, sensitivity to the holiness in the moment, simplicity of lifestyle, and the practice of communal spiritual relationships with those around us.[41] The contemplative way, James Finley asserts, does not involve striving for some distant goal, exploring obscure teaching, or embracing some unique meditation practices.[42] Becoming a person with a contemplative heart, a contemplative spirit, means becoming "one who spontaneously gravitates toward the depth of divinity manifested in each and every situation."[43]

I really don't think it's too difficult for we nurses to carry out contemplative caregiving by finding God in the practice of our profession. We do this often by seeing the presence of the Lord in our suffering patients, and in the life-and-death situations we experience daily. Our work is, by its very nature, attuned to seeking the presence of the Divine in its practice. We generally do well with communal relationships also; we need the support of like-minded others to carry on. As for simplicity of lifestyle, one might argue that the constraints of time and finances usually make that a given for nurses. And, in regard to sensitivity to the holiness in the moment, frequent and unanticipated crises have prepared us to lean on the Lord many times each day.

For me, however, the more difficult practice suggested for an aspiring contemplative has been that relating to "scheduled solitude"; it just hasn't seem to fit very well into my highly task-oriented schedule. To seek out a quiet time of prayerful solitude, although I have always been deeply aware of its value, has in the past appeared somewhat selfish; there always seemed so much need around me, so much work to do. When I verbalized that thought some years ago to a Franciscan Sister friend, she replied: "Don't forget the woman with the alabaster jar!"

The woman with the alabaster jar is described by all four evangelists as being greatly loved and honored by the Lord for her devotion and attention to Him. Matthew relates how, when Jesus was at Bethany, a woman poured an alabaster jar of costly perfume on his head while he reclined at table. When the disciples complained that the money spent for the perfume could have been given to the poor, Jesus replied, "The poor you will always have with you; but you will not always have me." He concluded by asserting that wherever the gospel was proclaimed "in the whole world," what the woman had done would be spoken of "in memory of her" (Matthew 26: 6–13).

Mark's account of the incident is very similar to that of Matthew; in Mark's story, however, the alabaster jar was broken. (Ancient alabaster flasks were often made without handles and with "a long neck that was broken to pour out the perfume."[44]) A note to Mark's gospel (Mark 14: 3–9) explains the importance of the woman's loving act of anointing Jesus in anticipation of His death; because Jesus would be crucified and buried as a criminal, his body would not have the usual preburial ritual of anointing.[45]

Luke interjects some different details into the narrative, reporting that Jesus was dining at the home of a pharisee when a sinful woman approached him with an alabaster flask. After bathing Jesus' feet with her tears and drying them with her hair, she anointed His feet with precious anointment. When the pharasee commented that Jesus, as a prophet, should know what sort of woman was touching him, Jesus taught him a parable of forgiveness. He explained that the woman had shown "great love" and so her "many sins" were forgiven (Luke 7: 36–49).

Finally, John suggests that it was Mary, the sister of Martha and Lazarus, who anointed Jesus' feet with "costly perfumed oil." In John's account, Judas, who would later betray Jesus, criticized Mary's "waste" of money. Jesus is again described as saying: "You always have the poor with you, but you do not always have me" (John 12: 1-8).

In exploring how one might become a "lay contemplative," Mary Frolich seems to also liken the concept of solitary contemplative prayer to the scriptural narrative of "the woman with the alabaster jar." She observes regarding meditative prayer: "This reckless pouring out of the precious ointment of time, combined with a constant and singlehearted focus on the beloved, is profoundly countercultural in today's world of tight schedules and short attention spans."[46] Frolich adds, however, that "One who submits regularly to the discipline of such a conversation will find a deeper, more attentive, more gentle self being shaped by it."[47]

The pondering of the woman with the alabaster jar scriptures has helped me understand that we nurses, as well as each being called by our founder to be a nurse "with a lamp," are each also called by the Lord to be a nurse "with an alabaster jar." To be compassionate caregivers, we must keep our hearts ever open and our lamps burning to light our path toward those in need. To be contemplative caregivers, we must never be afraid to "recklessly pour out the precious ointment" of our time in the presence of the Beloved. This is the secret of a contemplative life; this is the grace of contemplative caregiving. This is the blessing of becoming a "nurse with an alabaster jar."

THE PRAYER OF A CONTEMPLATIVE CAREGIVER

"I came so that they might have life and have it more abundantly."
John 10: 10

O God of magnificence and mystery, what must You be who gifted life with such beauty and such grace. Teach me to contemplate You, through tender care for the sacredness of all human life. Help me to revere the gifts of my ill brothers and sisters; to see in each person a reflection of Your face. Help me to love those I serve in their strengths and in their weaknesses; in caring for them, may I care for You, my Lord and my God. Let my nursing become an unceasing hymn of praise to Your glory, that I may pray with the psalmist:

"O Lord, our God, how awesome is Your Name through all the earth. What are humans that you are mindful of them; mere mortals that You care for them? Yet You have made them little less than a god; crowned them with glory and honor. You have given them rule over the works of Your hands, put all things under their feet ... O Lord, our God, how awesome is Your Name through all the earth" (Psalm 8). Amen.

Notes

CHAPTER 1: PRAYER IN NURSING: Reclaiming Our Spiritual Heritage

1. Mary Clare Vincent, *The Life of Prayer and the Way to God* (Petersham, Mass.: Saint Bede's Publications, 1982), 1.

2. Florence Nightingale, *Notes on Nursing: What It Is and What It Is Not* (London: Harrison, Bookseller to the Queen, 1859), 70–71.

3. Mary Elizabeth O'Brien, *Spirituality in Nursing: Standing on Holy Ground* (Sudbury, Mass.: Jones and Bartlett Publishers, 1999), 21–55.

4. Barbara M. Dossey, *Florence Nightingale: Mystic, Visionary, Healer* (Springhouse, Pa.: Springhouse Corporation, 2000), 33.

5. Ibid., 65.

6. Janet Macrae, "Nightingale's Spiritual Philosophy and Its Significance for Modern Nursing," *Image* 27:1 (1995): 10.

7. Dossey, 334.

8. Martha Vicinus and Bea Nergaard, *Ever Yours, Florence Nightingale: Selected Letters* (Cambridge, Mass.: Harvard University Press, 1990), 205.

9. Ibid.

10. Michael D. Calabria and Janet Macrae, *Suggestions for Thought by Florence Nightingale* (Philadelphia: University of Pennsylvania Press, 1994), 127.

11. Francis S. White, "At the Gate of the Temple," *The Public Health Nurse* 15:6 (1923): 283.

12. G. T. Lumpkin, "The Christ Spirit Which Makes the Hospital Great," *The Trained Nurse and Hospital Review* 77:6 (1926): 628.

13. "Mary's Nurse," *American Journal of Nursing* 29:12 (1929): 1445.

14. Ibid.

15. Ella L. Rothweiler, *The Science and Art of Nursing* (Philadelphia: F.A. Davis Company, 1937), 332.

16. William J. Thompson, "Nurse's Prayer at Graduation Exercises," *The Trained Nurse and Hospital Review*, 103:7 (1939): 15.

17. Mary Berenice Beck, *The Nurse: Handmaid of the Divine Physician* (Philadelphia: J.B. Lippincott Company, 1945), xvii.

18. Anthony Maher, "A Night Nurse's Prayer," *The Catholic Nurse*, 2:4 (1954): 30.

19. Edward J. Hayes, Paul J. Hayes, and Dorothy E. Kelly, *Moral Handbook of Nursing* (New York: The Macmillan Company, 1956), 134.

20. O'Brien, 1999, 108.

21. John H. Wright, "Prayer," in *The New Dictionary of Catholic Spirituality*, ed. Michael Downey (Collegeville, Minn.: The Liturgical Press, 1993), 764.

22. James M. Reese, "Prayer," in *The New Dictionary of Theology*, eds. Joseph Komonchak, Mary Collins, and Dermot Lane (Collegeville, Minn.: The Liturgical Press, 1990), 790.

23. Sandra S. Garant, *Living in Prayer* (Boston, Mass.: Pauline Books and Media, 1996), 9.

24. Arland J. Hultgren, "Prayer," in *Harper's Bible Dictionary*, ed. Paul J. Achtemeier (San Francisco: Harper & Row, Publishers, 1985), 816.

25. Barbara Fiand, *Releasement: Spirituality in Ministry* (New York: Crossroad, 1991), 88–89.

26. Maureen Conroy, *The Discerning Heart: Discovering a Personal God* (Chicago: Loyola Press, 1993), 198.

27. William A. Barry, *Discernment in Prayer: Paying Attention to God* (Notre Dame, In.: Ave Maria Press, 1990), 21.

28. William J. Rademacher, *Lay Ministry: A Theological, Spiritual and Pastoral Handbook* (New York: Crossroad, 1991), 201–202.

29. Brother Roger of Taize, *No Greater Love* (Collegeville, Minn.: The Liturgical Press, 1991), 8.

30. Edward J. Malatesta, "Charism," in *The New Dictionary of Catholic Spirituality*, ed. Michael Downey (Collegeville, Minn.: The Liturgical Press, 1993), 140.

31. Peter M. Stravinskas, ed., *Our Sunday Visitor Catholic Encyclopedia* (Huntington, In.: Our Sunday Visitor, Inc., 1998), 223.

32. Gerald O'Collins and Edward G. Farrugia, *A Concise Dictionary of Theology* (Mahwah, N.J.: Paulist Press, 2000), 40.

33. John L. Gillman, "Charism," in *The Collegeville Pastoral Dictionary of Biblical Theology* (Collegeville, Minn.: The Liturgical Press, 1996), 128.

34. Susan Muto, *Catholic Spirituality from A to Z: An Inspirational Dictionary* (Ann Arbor, Mi.: Servant Publications, 2000), 40.

35. Richard P. McBrian, ed., *The HarperCollins Encyclopedia of Catholicism* (San Francisco: HarperSanFrancisco, 1995), 300.

36. Muto, 68.

37. Francis De Sales, *Introduction to a Devout Life*, trans. and ed. John K. Ryan (New York: Image Books, 1989), 44.

38. Carl Dehne, "Devotion," in *The New Dictionary of Theology*, eds. Joseph Komonchak, Mary Collins, and Dermot Lane (Collegeville, Minn.: The Liturgical Press, 1990), 283.

39. Benedict Groeschel, "Introduction," in *In the Presence of Our Lord*, eds. Benedict Groeschel and James Monti (Huntington, In.: Our Sunday Visitor Publishing Division, 1997), 15.

40. Monica Baly, ed., *As Miss Nightingale Said ... Florence Nightingale Through Her Sayings: A Victorian Perspective* (London: Scutari Press, 1991), 68.

41. Florence Nightingale, *Notes on Nursing: What It Is and What It Is Not* (London: Harrison, 1859), 70.

42. Baly, 19.

43. Susan Cahill, ed., *Wise Women: Over Two Thousand Years of Spiritual Writing by Women* (New York: W.W. Norton & Company, 1996), 143.

44. M. Adelaide Nutting and Lavinia L. Dock, *A History of Nursing*, Vol. 2 (New York: G.P. Putnam's Sons, 1935), 116.

45. Ibid.

46. Anne L. Austin, ed., *History of Nursing Sourcebook* (New York: G.P. Putnam's Sons, 1957), 236.

47. Minnie Goodnow, *Outlines of Nursing History* (Philadelphia: W.B. Saunders Company, 1916), 56.

48. Edward F. Garesche, *Ethics and the Art of Conduct for Nurses* (Philadelphia: W.B. Saunders Company, 1929), 258.

49. Ibid., 259.

50. Joseph F. Power, *Francis De Sales: Finding God Wherever You Are* (Hyde Park, N.Y.: New City Press, 1993), 35.

51. Jean-Pierre De Caussade, *Abandonment to Divine Providence*, trans. John Beevers (New York: Image Books, 1975), 42.

52. Brother Lawrence of the Resurrection, *Writings and Conversations on the Practice of the Presence of God*, ed. Conrad Meester and trans. Salvatore Sciurba (Washington, D.C.: Institute of Carmelite Studies, 1994), xxxv.

53. Ibid.

54. Carlo Carretto, *Summoned by Love* (Maryknoll, N.Y.: Orbis Books, 1978), 76.

CHAPTER 2. A HOLY CALLING: Prayer and Commitment to Nursing

1. *The Catholic Nurse*, 3:3 (1955), 36.

2. Lawrence S. Cunningham, "Holiness," in *The New Dictionary of Catholic Spirituality*, ed. Michael Downey (Collegeville, Minn.: Liturgical Press, 1993), 479.

3. Mary Elizabeth O'Brien, *The Nurse's Calling: A Christian Spirituality of Caring for the Sick* (Mahwah, N.J.: Paulist Press, 2001).

4. Joyce Rupp, *May I Have This Dance?* (Notre Dame, In.: Ave Maria Press, 1992), 117.

5. *The Call of Silent Love* (Kalamazoo, Mi.: Cistercian Publications, 1995), 32.

6. Barbara Dossey, *Florence Nightingale: Mystic, Visionary and Healer* (Springhouse, Pa.: Springhouse Corporation, 2000), 3.

7. Madeleine C. Vaillot, *Commitment to Nursing: A Philosophic Investigation* (Philadelphia, Pa.: J.B. Lippincott Company, 1962), 13.

8. Ibid.

9. Eleanor A. Tourtillott, *Commitment: A Lost Characteristic* (New York: National League for Nursing, 1982), 13.

10. Verna Benner Carson, "Spirituality and the Nursing Process," in *Spiritual Dimensions of Nursing Practice*, ed. Verna Carson (Philadelphia, Pa.: W.B. Saunders Company, 1989), 168.

11. Ibid.

12. Robert P. Maloney C.M., *The Way of Vincent de Paul: A Contemporary Spirituality in the Service of the Poor* (New Rochelle, N.Y.: New City Press, 1992), 37.

13. Lena D. Dietz and Aurelia R. Lehosky, *History and Modern Nursing* (Philadelphia: F.A. Davis Company, 1967), 189–190.

14. Ibid., 190.

15. Minnie Goodnow, *Nursing History* (Philadelphia: W.B. Saunders Company, 1948), 12.

16. Judith Calhoun, "The Nightingale Pledge: A Commitment that Survives the Passage of Time," *Nursing and Health Care* 14:3 (1993), 130–136.

17. Beth McBurney and Tina Filoromo, "The Nightingale Pledge: 100 Years Later," *Nursing Management* 25:2 (1994), 74.

18. Teresa Betts-Cobau and Paulette Hoyer, "Domestic Violence: Are Professional Pledges Such as the Nightingale Pledge Obsolete?" *Journal of Perinatal Education* 6:4 (1997): 17–27, 37–38.

19. Maloney, 53.

20. McBurney and Filoromo, 72.

21. Joseph A. Bracken, "Community," in *The New Dictionary of Theology*, eds. Joseph Komonchak, Mary Collins, and Dermot Lane (Collegeville, Minn.: The Liturgical Press, 1990), 216.

22. Bernard J. Lee, "Community," in *The New Dictionary of Catholic Spirituality*, ed. Michael Downey (Collegeville, Minn.: The Liturgical Press, 1993), 184.

23. Michael Casey, "Apatheia," in Downey, 50.

24. Helen Doohan, "Beatitudes," in Downey, 81–82.

25. Ibid, 82.

26. Margaret Eckert, "Ethics and Values," in *Fundamentals of Nursing*, 5th ed., eds. Patrice A. Potter and Anne G. Perry (St. Louis, Mo.: Mosby, 2001), 404.

27. Carol Taylor, Carol Lillis, and Priscilla LeMone, *Fundamentals of Nursing: The Art and Science of Nursing Care* (Philadelphia, Pa.: J.B. Lippincott Company, 2001), 84.

28. Ibid.

29. Calhoun, 134.

30. Potter and Perry (Eckert), 410.

31. Taylor, Lillis, and LeMone, 82.

32. Ibid.

33. Taylor, Lillis, and LeMone, 320.

34. Judith Wilkinson, "Values, Ethics and Advocacy," in *Fundamentals of Nursing: Concepts, Process and Practice*, eds. Barbara Kozier, Glenora Erb, Audrey Berman, and Karen Burke (Upper Saddle River, N.J.: Prentice Hall Health, 2000), 77.

35. Ibid, 78.

36. Monica Baly, ed., *As Miss Nightingale Said ... Florence Nightingale Through Her Sayings: A Victorian Perspective* (London: Scutari Press, 1991), 68.

37. William J. Rademacher, *Lay Ministry: A Theological, Spiritual and Pastoral Handbook* (New York: Crossroad, 1991), 196.

CHAPTER 3: OPENNESS TO THE SPIRIT: Prayer and Becoming a Vessel

1. Margery Williams, *The Velveteen Rabbit* (New York: Avon Books, 1975), 13.

2. Thomas R.W. Longstaff, "The Holy Spirit," in *Harper's Bible Dictionary*, ed. Paul J. Achtemeier (San Francisco: Harper & Row, Publishers, 1985), 401.

3. Robert P. Imbelli, "Holy Spirit," in *The New Dictionary of Theology*, eds. Joseph A. Komonchak, Mary Collins, and Dermot Lane (Collegeville, Minn.: The Liturgical Press, 1990), 488.

4. M. John Farrelly, "Holy Spirit," in *The New Dictionary of Catholic Spirituality*, ed. Michael Downey (Collegeville, Minn.: The Liturgical Press, 1993), 492.

5. Elizabeth A. Livingstone, ed., *The Concise Oxford Dictionary of the Christian Church* (New York: Oxford University Press, 1990), 245.

6. *The Call of Silent Love* (Kalamazoo, Mi.: Cistercian Publications, 1995), 89.

7. Mark Thibodeaux, *Armchair Mystic: Easing Into Contemplative Prayer* (Cincinnati, Ohio: St. Anthony Messenger Press, 2001), 17–28.

8. Ibid, 73–74.

9. Benedict J. Groeschel, *Listening at Prayer* (New York: Paulist Press, 1984), 12–15.

10. David Lonsdale, *Listening to the Music of the Spirit: The Art of Discernment* (Notre Dame, In.: Ave Maria Press, 1992), 45.

11. Maureen Conroy, *The Discerning Heart: Discovering a Personal God* (Chicago: Loyola Press, 1993), xi.

12. Thomas H. Green, *Opening to God* (Notre Dame, In.: Ave Maria Press, 1998), 45, 47.

13. Gerald May, *The Awakened Heart* (San Francisco: HarperSanFrancisco, 1991), 121–122.

14. Peter Kreeft, *Prayer for Beginners* (San Francisco: Ignatius Press, 2000), 34.

15. Page Zyromski, *Pray the Bible* (Cincinnati, Ohio: St. Anthony Messenger Press, 2000).

16. Groeschel, 1984.

17. Michael Casey, *Toward God: The Ancient Wisdom of Western Prayer* (Liguori, Mo.: Liguori/Triumph, 1996.

18. William A. Barry, *God and You: Prayer as a Personal Relationship* (New York: Paulist Press, 1987).

19. *Collegeville Series on Books of the Bible* (Collegeville, Minn.: Liturgical Press, 1987).

20. Pierre Wolff, *The Hungry Heart* (Liguori, Mo.: Triumph Books, 1995), 7.

21. Ibid, 7–10.

22. Barbara M. Dossey, *Florence Nightingale: Mystic, Visionary, Healer* (Springhouse, Pa.: Springhouse Corporation, 2000), 338.

23. Mary Berenice Beck, *The Nurse: Handmaid of the Divine Physician* (Philadelphia: J.B. Lippincott Company, 1945), 248.

24. Kamalini Kumar, "Work as Worship," *Journal of Christian Nursing* 16:2 (1999), 9.

CHAPTER 4. A SACRED COVENANT: Prayer and the Nurse-Patient Relationship

1. Mary Elizabeth O'Brien, *The Nurse's Calling: A Christian Spirituality of Caring for the Sick* (Mahwah, N.J.: Paulist Press, 2001), 20.

2. Mary Elizabeth O'Brien, *Spirituality in Nursing: Standing on Holy Ground* (Sudbury, Mass.: Jones and Bartlett Publishers, 1999); Mary Elizabeth O'Brien, *The Nurse's Calling: A Christian Spirituality of Caring for the Sick* (Mahwah, N.J.: Paulist Press, 2001).

3. O'Brien, 1999, 86.

4. Irene Nowell, "Covenant," in *The New Dictionary of Theology*, eds. Joseph Komonchak, Mary Collins, and Dermot Lane (Collegeville, Minn.: The Liturgical Press, 1990), 243.

5. Donald Senior, "Covenant," in *The New Dictionary of Catholic Spirituality*, ed. Michael Downey (Collegeville, Minn.: The Liturgical Press, 1993), 237.

6. Mary C. Cooper, "Covenental Relationships: Grounding for the Nursing Ethic," *Advances in Nursing Science* 10:4 (1988): 50.

7. M. Manning, "Together: Let's Keep Our Covenant to Care," *Massachusetts Nurse* 67:4 (1997), 3.

8. Judith B. Krauss, "The Nurse-Patient Covenant and the Imperative to Care," *Archives of Psychiatric Nursing*, 12:6 (1998): 299.

9. Richard Foster, *Prayer: Finding the Heart's True Home* (San Francisco: HarperSanFrancisco, 1992), 70.

10. Simon Tugwell, *Prayer: Living with God* (Springfield, Ill.: Templegate Publishers, 1975), vii.

11. Foster, 70.

12. William Barry, *Discernment in Prayer: Paying Attention to God* (Notre Dame, In.: Ave Maria Press, 1990), 17.

13. Joan Chittister, *The Rule of Benedict: Insight for the Ages* (New York: Crossroad, 1998), 99–100.

14. Verna Benner Carson, "The Nurse-Patient Relationship," in *Fundamentals of Nursing: Collaborating for Optimal Health*, 2nd ed., eds. Karen J. Berger and Marilyn B. Williams (Stamford, Ct.: Appleton & Lange, 1999), 286.

15. Janet Brown, "Caring, Comforting and Communicating," in *Fundamentals of Nursing: Concepts, Process and Practice*, 6th ed., eds. Barbara Kozier, Glenora Erb, Audrey Berman, and Karen Burke (Upper Saddle River, N.J.: Prentice Hall Health, 2000), 439.

16. Daria Virvan, "The Nurse-Client Relationship," in *Fundamentals of Nursing, Caring and Clinical Judgement*, ed. Helen Harkreader (Philadelphia, Pa.: W.B. Saunders Company, 2000), 307.

17. Joseph J. Schmidt, *Praying Our Experiences* (Winnona, Minn.: Saint Mary's Press, 2000), 70.

18. Corita Clarke, *A Spirituality for Active Ministry* (Kansas City, Mo.: Sheed & Ward, 1991), 26.

19. Claude Morel, *15 Days of Prayer with Saint Francis De Sales* (Liguori, Mo.: Liguori Publications, 2000), 33.

20. Brother Lawrence of the Resurrection, *The Practice of the Presence of God* (Mount Vernon, N.Y.: Peter Pauper Press, 1973), 48.

21. Jean-Pierre De Caussade, *Abandonment to Divine Providence*, trans. John Beevers (New York: Image Books, 1975), 23.

22. Ignatius Loyola cited in William A. Barry, *What Do I Want in Prayer?* (New York: Paulist Press, 1994), 119.

23. *Clinical Journal of Oncology Nursing* 4:3 (May/June 2000).

24. Pamela J. Lewis, "A Review of Prayer within the Role of the Holistic Nurse, *Journal of Holistic Nursing* 14:4 (1996), 308–315.

25. J. Mauk, "Spirituality Through Centering Prayer in School Nursing," *Journal of School Nursing* 14:2 (1998): 49–51.

26. M. Holt-Ashley, "Nurses Pray: Use of Prayer and Spirituality as a Complementary Therapy in the Intensive Care Setting," *AACN Clinical Issues: Advanced Practice in Acute and Critical Care*, 11:1 (2000): 60–67.

27. S.C. Sellers and B.A. Haag, "Spiritual Nursing Interventions," *Journal of Holistic Nursing* 16: 3 (1998): 338–354.

28. Carolyn H. Mason, "Prayer as a Nursing Intervention," *Journal of Christian Nursing* 12:1 (1995): 4–8; Judith Shelly and Sharon Fish, "Praying with Patients," *Journal of Christian Nursing* 12:1 (1995): 9–13.

29. Pierre Wolff, *The Hungry Heart* (Liguori, Mo.: Triumph Books, 1995), 96.

30. Mary Clare Vincent, *The Life of Prayer and the Way to God* (Petersham, Mass.: Saint Bede's Publications, 1981), 44.

31. Abraham Heschel, *The Sabbath: Its Meaning for Modern Man* (New York: Ferrar, Straus and Giroux, 1979), 13.

32. Ibid., 10.

CHAPTER 5: COMPASSIONATE CAREGIVING: Prayer and Embracing Patients' Needs

1. Frederick J. Rosenheim, "Captives of God," *The Catholic Nurse* 3:2 (1954): 29.

2. Wayne Simsic, *Songs of Sunrise, Seeds of Prayer* (Mystic, Ct.: Twenty-Third Publications, 1991), 75.

3. Brother Roger of Taize, *His Love Is a Fire* (Collegeville, Minn.: The Liturgical Press, 1990), 32.

4. Henri Nouwen, *Reaching Out: The Three Movements of the Spiritual Life* (New York: Image Books, 1975), 136.

5. *The Wound of Love: A Carthusian Miscellaney* (Kalamazoo, Mi.: Cistercian Publications, 1994), 70.

6. L. Kacperek, "Non-Verbal Communication: The Importance of Listening," *British Journal of Nursing* 6:5 (1997): 13–26.

7. K.C. King, "Using Therapeutic Silence in Home Healthcare Nursing," *Home Health Nurse* 13:1 (1995): 65–68.

8. John Cardinal O'Connor, *A Moment of Grace: John Cardinal O'Connor on the Catechism of the Catholic Church* (San Francisco: Ignatius Press, 1995), 214.

9. Jerome Kodell, *The Gospel According to Luke* (Collegeville, Minn.: The Liturgical Press, 1989), 7.

10. Adrian Van Kaam, *Spirituality and the Gentle Life* (Denville, N.Y.: Dimension Books Inc., 1974), 19.

11. Ibid., 28.

12. Judith Lechman, *The Spirituality of Gentleness* (San Francisco: Harper & Row Publishers, 1989), 1.

13. Joseph F. Power, *Francis De Sales: Finding God Wherever You Are* (Hyde Park, N.Y.: New City Press, 1993), 34.

14. Harrison A. Williams, "Gentleness," *Theology* 65:1 (1962): 355.

15. Don Hill, *Life by Design* (Danville, Ky.: Lay Leadership International, 1994), 49.

16. Robert Strand, *Nine Fruits of the Spirit: Gentleness* (Green Forest, Ark.: New Leaf Press, 1999), 35.

17. Joseph C. Aldrich, *Gentle Persuasion: Creative Ways to Introduce Your Friends to Christ* (Portland, Ore.: Multnomah, 1988), 75.

18. Phyllis J. LePeau, *Gentleness, the Strength of Being Tender* (Grand Rapids, Mi.: Zondervan Publishing House, 1991), 1.

19. Anthony J. Ciorra, *Everyday Mysticism: Cherishing the Holy* (New York: Crossroad, 1996), 133–134.

20. Annie L. Austin, ed., *History of Nursing Sourcebook* (New York: G.P. Putnam's Sons, 1957), 254.

21. Florence Nightingale, *Notes on Nursing: What It Is and What It Is Not* (London: Harrison, Bookseller to the Queen, 1859), 28.

22. Clara Weeks-Shaw, *A Textbook of Nursing*, 2nd ed. (New York: D. Appleton and Company, 1892), 12.

23. Isabel A. Hampton, ed., *Nursing of the Sick* (New York: McGraw-Hill Book Company, Inc., 1893), 34.

24. T. Billroth, *The Care of the Sick at Home and in the Hospital*, trans. J. Bentall Endean (London: Sampson, Low, Marston and Company, Ltd., 1895), 21.

25. Emily A. Strong, *Practical Points in Nursing* (Philadelphia, Pa.: W.B. Saunders, 1898), 19.

26. Isabel H. Robb, *Nursing Ethics: For Hospital and Private Use* (Cleveland, Ohio: C.C. Koeckert Publishers, 1919), 81–82.

27. Charlotte A. Aikens, *Studies in Ethics for Nurses* (Philadelphia, Pa.: W.B. Saunders Company, 1928), 43.

28. Virginia D. Homans, "A Nurse's Prayer," *American Journal of Nursing* 29:8 (1929): 1028.

29. Walter Rauschenbauch, "A Prayer for Doctors and Nurses," *American Journal of Nursing* 29:8 (1929): 943.

30. Katherine Shephard and Charles H. Lawrence, *Textbook of Attendant Nursing* (New York: The Macmillan Company, 1935), 366.

31. Raymond Hain, "Capping Exercises," *The Catholic Nurse* 3:1 (1954): 57.

32. Sr. Evangela, "Poem on Geriatrics," *The Catholic Nurse* 17:3 (1969): 31.

33. Jean Hayter, "Patients Who Have Alzheimer's Disease," *American Journal of Nursing* 74:8 (1974): 1460–1463.

34. Jeanne M. McNally, "Gentleness: An Attribute for Administrators," *Supervisor Nurse* 7:10 (1976): 70–71.

35. Lori Carley, "Reaching Julie with a Gentle Touch," *Nursing '87* 17:2 (1987): 38–40.

36. Dominic Chung, "The Gentle Touch ... Could We, Should We?" *Nursing Times* 77:7 (1981): 287–290.

37. Julia Keachie, "Gentle Persuasion," *Nursing Times* 88:6 (1992): 40.

38. K. Kirk, "Chronically Ill Patients: Perceptions of Nursing Care," *Rehabilitation Nursing* 18:2 (1993): 99–104.

39. A. Scott, "Patients' Perceptions of Openness in Nurses: A Strategic Ethnography," *Journal of Theory Construction and Testing* 1:2 (1997): 40–45.

40. J.R. Boyd and M. Hunsberger, "Chronically Ill Children Coping with Repeated Hospitalizations," *Journal of Pediatric Nursing* 13:6 (1998): 330–342.

CHAPTER 6: THE WOUNDED HEALER: Prayer and the Problem of Suffering

1. William A. Barry, *God and You: Prayer as a Personal Relationship* (New York: Paulist Press, 1987), 47.

2. Simon Tugwell, *Prayer in Practice* (Springfield, Ill.: Templegate Publishers, 1974), 45.

3. Dennis Billy, *Soliloquy Prayer: Unfolding Our Hearts to God* (Liguori, Mo.: Liguori Publications, 1998), 54.

4. Max Oliva, *Free to Pray, Free to Love* (Notre Dame, In.: Ave Maria Press, 1994), 74.

5. Jacqueline Bergan and Marie Schwan, *Surrender: A Guide for Prayer* (Winona, Minn.: Saint Mary's Press, 1986), 10.

6. Pierre Wolff, *The Hungry Heart* (Liguori, Mo.: Triumph Books, 1995), 90–91.

7. Peter Kreeft, *Prayer for Beginners* (San Francisco: Ignatius Press, 2000), 77.

8. Oliva, 87.

9. Thomas H. Green, *When the Well Runs Dry: Prayer Beyond the Beginnings* (Notre Dame, In.: Ave Maria Press, 1998), 123.

10. Ibid., 81.

11. Mary Clare Vincent, *The Life of Prayer and the Way to God* (Petersham, Mass.: Saint Bede's Publications, 1982), 67.

12. Ibid., 67.

13. Green, 105.

14. Richard J. Foster, *Prayer: Finding the Heart's True Home* (San Francisco: Harper-SanFrancisco, 1992), 181.

15. Ibid., 182–183.

16. Wolff, 123.

17. Mary Elizabeth O'Brien, *Spirituality in Nursing: Standing on Holy Ground* (Sudbury, Mass.: Jones and Bartlett Publishers, 1999); Mary Elizabeth O'Brien, *The Nurse's Calling: A Christian Spirituality of Caring for the Sick* (Mahwah, N.J.: Paulist Press, 2000).

18. O'Brien, 1999, 64.

19. Lucy Ridgely Seymer, ed., *Selected Writings of Florence Nightingale* (New York: The Macmillan Company, 1954), 351.

20. "France's Heroine: 'Catholic Nurse,'" *The Catholic Nurse* 3:1 (1954): 47.

CHAPTER 7: THE JOURNEY TO JERUSALEM: Prayer and a Healing Ministry

1. Jerome Kodell, *The Gospel According to Luke* (Collegeville, Minn.: The Liturgical Press, 1989), 57.

2. Benedict Groeschel, *Listening at Prayer* (Mahwah, N.J.: Paulist Press, 1984).

3. Mary E. Heyward, "The Golden Jubilee at the Catholic University School of Nursing," *The Trained Nurse and Hospital Review* 11:4 (1939): 346.

4. "The Nurse's Mass," *The Catholic Nurse* 2:2 (1953): 54.

5. Matthew Miller, "Modern Veronicas," *The Catholic Nurse* 2:3 (1954): 20.

6. W.L. Hawley, "The Lay Apostolate in Nursing," *The Catholic Nurse* 2:3 (1954): 17.

7. Albert G. Meyer, "The Catholic Nurse: A Modern Veronica," *The Catholic Nurse* 7:1 (1958): 47.

8. Ibid., 47, 56.

9. Eileen Ridgway, "Veronica," *The Catholic Nurse* 8:3 (1960): 67.

10. Sr. Marie George, "A Way of the Cross for Nurses," *The Catholic Nurse* 12:3 (1964): 57.

11. Josephine Dolan, *Nursing in Society: A Historical Perspective* (Philadelphia: W.B. Saunders Company, 1973), 49.

12. Wilhelm Schneemelcher, ed., *Edgar Hennecke: New Testament Apocrypha*, Vol. 1 (Philadelphia: The Westminster Press, 1963), 457.

13. B. Harris Cowper, *The Apocryphal Gospels and Other Documents Relating to the History of Christ* (London: David Nutt, 1897), 224.

14. Alvin E. Ford, ed., *La Vengeance de Nostre Seigneur* (Toronto, Ontario: Pontifical Institute of Mediaeval Studies, 1984), 6.

15. Elizabeth A. Livingstone, *The Concise Oxford Dictionary of the Christian Church* (New York: Oxford University Press, 1999), 530.

16. T. Ronald Haney, *Stations of the Cross: The Story of God's Compassion* (New York: Crossroad, 1999), 36.

17. Herbert J. Thurston and Donald Attwater, eds., *Butler's Lives of the Saints*, Vol. 2 (Allen, Tx.: Thomas More Publishing, 1996), 83.

18. Robert Ellsberg, *All Saints: Daily Reflections on Saints, Prophets and Witnesses for Our Time* (New York: Crossroad, 1998), 299.

19. Matthew Bunson, Margaret Bunson, and Stephen Bunson, *Our Sunday Visitor's Encyclopedia of Saints* (Huntington, In.: Our Sunday Visitor Inc., 1998), 633.

20. Nicholas Ayo, James Flanigan, Joseph Ross, and J.M. Ford, *Where Joy and Sorrow Meet: A Way of the Cross* (Notre Dame, In.: Ave Maria Press, 1999), 78–79.

21. Margaret Bunson and Matthew Bunson, *Lives of the Saints You Should Know*, Vol. 2 (Huntington, In.: Our Sunday Visitor Inc., 1996), 158.

22. Ellsberg, 299.

23. Caryll Houselander, *The Way of the Cross* (New York: Sheed & Ward, 1955), 69.

24. Ibid., 70.

25. Florence Nightingale, *Notes on Nursing: What It Is and What It Is Not* (London: Harrison and Sons, 1859), 53.

26. Ibid., 53.

27. Isabel Hampton Robb, *Nursing: Its Principles and Practice* (Cleveland, Ohio: E.C. Koeckert Publisher, 1906), 138.

28. Amy Elizabeth Pope and Virna M. Young, *The Art and Principles of Nursing* (New York: G.P. Putnam's Sons, 1934), 85.

29. Bertha Harmer and Virginia Henderson, *Textbook of the Principles and Practice of Nursing* (New York: The Macmillan Company, 1939), 286.

30. Alice L. Price, *The Art and Science of Nursing* (Philadelphia: W.B. Saunders Company, 1954), 173.

31. Virginia Henderson and Gladys Nite, *Principles and Practice of Nursing* (New York: Macmillan Publishing Company, 1978), 789.

32. Helen Harkreader, *Fundamentals of Nursing: Caring and Clinical Judgement* (Philadelphia: W.B. Saunders, 2000), 927.

33. Joyce Rupp, *Fresh Bread and Other Gifts of Spiritual Nourishment* (Notre Dame, In.: Ave Maria Press, 1993), 31–32.

34. Suzanne Gorden, *Life Support: Three Nurses on the Front Lines* (Boston: Little Brown and Company, 1997).

35. Ibid., 19.

36. Ibid., 19.

37. Ibid., 19.

38. Mary Elizabeth O'Brien, *Spirituality in Nursing: Standing on Holy Ground* (Sudbury, Mass.: Jones and Bartlett Publishers, 1999).

39. Mary Elizabeth O'Brien, *The Nurse's Calling: A Christian Spirituality of Caring for the Sick* (Mahwah, N.J.: Paulist Press, 2001).

40. Livingstone, 270–271.

41. Bruce E. Schein, "Jerusalem," in *Harper's Bible Dictionary*, ed. Paul J. Achtemeier (San Francisco: Harper & Row Publishers, 1985), 465.

42. Daniel J. Harrington, *The Gospel According to Matthew* (Collegeville, Minn.: The Liturgical Press, 1991), 85.

43. Philip Van Linden, *The Gospel According to Mark* (Collegeville, Minn.: The Liturgical Press, 1991), 65.

44. Kodell, 96.

45. Neal M. Flanigan, *The Gospel According to John and the Johannine Epistles* (Collegeville, Minn.: The Liturgical Press, 1989), 55.

46. William H. Shannon, "Humility," in *The New Dictionary of Catholic Spirituality*, ed. Michael Downey (Collegeville, Minn.: The Liturgical Press, 1993), 516.

47. Ibid., 517.

48. Ibid., 517.

49. Nightingale, 71.

50. Carol Frances Jegen, "Peace," in *The New Catholic Dictionary of Spirituality*, ed. Michael Downey (Collegeville, Minn.: The Liturgical Press, 1993), 732–733.

51. Ibid., 733.

52. O'Brien, 1999, 179.

53. O'Brien, 1999, 26.

54. Helen Doohan, "Service," in *The New Catholic Dictionary of Spirituality*, ed. Michael Downey (Collegeville, Minn.: The Liturgical Press, 1993), 875.

55. Francis Schussler-Fiorenza, "Redemption," in *The New Dictionary of Theology*, eds. Joseph A. Komonchak, Mary Collins, and Dermot Lane (Collegeville, Minn.: The Liturgical Press), 836–837.

CHAPTER 8: THE ART OF CONTEMPLATIVE CAREGIVING

1. William A. Barry, *God and You: Prayer as Personal Relationship* (New York: Paulist Press, 1987), 57.

2. Thomas H. Green, *Opening to God: A Guide to Prayer* (Notre Dame, In.: Ave Maria Press, 1998), 86–87.

3. Peter Kreeft, *Prayer for Beginners* (San Francisco: Ignatius Press, 2000), 49–50.

4. Ibid., 27.

5. Pierre Wolff, *The Hungry Heart* (Liguori, Mo.: Triumph Books, 1995), 38.

6. Bartholomew J. O'Brien, *Primer on Prayer* (Milford, Ohio: Faith Publishing Company, 1991), 54.

7. Laurence Freeman, "Meditation," in *The New Dictionary of Catholic Spirituality*, ed. Michael Downey (Collegeville, Minn.: The Liturgical Press, 1993), 648.

8. James Finley, *The Contemplative Heart* (Notre Dame, In.: Sorin Books, 2000), 51.

9. Richard J. Foster, *Prayer: Finding the Heart's True Home* (San Francisco: HarperSanFrancisco, 1992), 143.

10. Michael Casey, *Toward God: The Ancient Wisdom of Western Prayer* (Liguori, Mo.: Liguori/Triumph, 1996), 105.

11. Joyce Huggett, *Learning the Language of Prayer* (New York: Crossroad, 1997), 37.

12. Jean-Marie Howe, *Spiritual Journey: The Monastic Way* (Petersham, Mass.: St. Bede's Publications, 1989), 67, 69.

13. Thelma Hall, *Too Deep for Words: Rediscovering Lectio Divina* (Mahwah, N.J.: Paulist Press, 1988), 28.

14. Andre Louf, *The Cistercian Way* (Kalamazoo, Mi.: Cistercian Publications, 1989), 75.

15. M. Basil Pennington, *Lectio Divina: Renewing the Ancient Practice of Praying the Scriptures* (New York: Crossroad, 1998), 32.

16. Thomas Keating, "Centering Prayer," in *The New Dictionary of Catholic Spirituality*, ed. Michael Downey (Collegeville, Minn.: The Liturgical Press, 1993), 139.

17. Ibid., 139.

18. William H. Shannon, "Contemplation, Contemplative Prayer," in *The New Dictionary of Catholic Spirituality*, ed. Michael Downey (Collegeville, Minn.: The Liturgical Press, 1993), 209.

19. *The Sermons of Saint Francis De Sales On Prayer*, ed. Lewis S. Fiorelli (Rockford, Ill.: Tan Books and Publishers, Inc., 1985), 3.

20. Brother Roger of Taize, *His Love Is a Fire* (Collegeville, Minn.: The Liturgical Press, 1990), 49.

21. Thomas Keating, *Invitation to Love: The Way of Christian Contemplation* (New York: Continuum, 1999), 145.

22. Morton Kelsey, *Spiritual Living in a Material World* (Hyde Park, N.Y.: New City Press, 1998), 49.

23. Duncan Basil, *Eyes on The Lord: View of a Contemplative* (Middlegreen, Slough, U.K.: St. Pauls, 1994), 77.

24. Hall, 2.

25. Foster, 159.

26. Mary Clare Vincent, *The Life of Prayer and The Way to God* (Petersham, Mass.: St. Bede's Publications, 1982), 73.

27. Wendy M. Wright, "Lay Contemplative Formation Programs," in *The Lay Contemplative*, eds. Virginia Manss and Mary Frohlich (Cincinnati, Ohio: St. Anthony Messenger Press, 2000), 91.

28. Ibid., 94.

29. Jacqueline Bergan and Marie Schwan, *Surrender: A Guide for Prayer* (Winona, Minn.: Saint Mary's Press, 1986), 5.

30. Wolff, 59.

31. Bergan and Schwan, 5.

32. Joseph F. Schmidt, *Praying Our Experiences* (Winona, Minn.: Saint Mary's Press, 2000), 42.

33. Mark E. Thibodeaux, *Armchair Mystic: Easing into Contemplative Prayer* (Cincinnati, Ohio: St. Anthony Messenger Press, 2001), 112.

34. John Welch, "Mysticism," in *The New Dictionary of Theology*, eds. Joseph Komonchak, Mary Collins, and Dermot Lane (Collegeville, Minn.: Liturgical Press, 1990), 694.

35. Ibid., 694–695.

36. James A. Wiseman, "Mysticism," in *The New Dictionary of Catholic Spirituality*, ed. Michael Downey (Collegeville, Minn.: The Liturgical Press, 1993), 692.

37. Mary Elizabeth O'Brien, *Spirituality in Nursing: Standing on Holy Ground* (Sudbury, Mass.: Jones and Bartlett Publishers, 1999), 115.

38. H.D. Egan, "The Mysticism of Everyday Life," *Studies in Formative Spirituality* 10:1 (1989): 8.

39. Ibid., 8.

40. Peggy Wilkenson, *Finding the Mystic within You* (Washington, D.C.: ICS Publications, 1999), 23.

41. Stephen K. Hatch, "The Formation of the Everyday Contemplative," in *The Lay Contemplative*, eds. Virginia Manss and Mary Frohlich (Cincinnati, Ohio: St. Anthony Messenger Press, 2000), 61–67.

42. James Finley, *The Contemplative Heart* (Notre Dame, In.: Sorin Books, 2000), 25.

43. Ibid., 29.

44. Paul J. Achtemeier, ed., *Harper's Bible Dictionary* (San Francisco: Harper & Row Publishers, 1985), 19.

45. Donald Senior, Mary Ann Getty, Carroll Stuhlmueller, and John Collins, eds., *The Catholic Study Bible: New American Bible* (New York: Oxford University Press, 1990), 89.

46. Mary Frohlich, "Contemplative Conversations with the 'Other,'" in *The Lay Contemplative: Testimonies, Perspectives, Resources*, eds. Virginia Manss and Mary Frohlich (Cincinnati, Ohio: St. Anthony Messenger Press, 2000), 78.

47. Ibid., 78.

Index